NEW PANDEMICS, OLD POLITICS

To my mother, Esther de Waal,
who taught me how to think.

NEW PANDEMICS, OLD POLITICS

Two Hundred Years of War on Disease and its Alternatives

Alex de Waal

polity

First published in 2021 by Polity Press

Polity Press
65 Bridge Street
Cambridge CB2 1UR, UK

Polity Press
101 Station Landing
Suite 300
Medford, MA 02155, USA

ISBN-13: 978-1-5095-4779-1
ISBN-13: 978-1-5095-4780-7 (pb)

A catalogue record for this book is available from the British Library.

Library of Congress Cataloging-in-Publication Data
Names: De Waal, Alex, author.
Title: New pandemics, old politics : two hundred years of war on disease and its alternatives / Alex de Waal.
Description: Medford : Polity Press, 2021. | Includes bibliographical references and index. | Summary: "A brilliant account of the politics behind modern pandemics by a leading expert on humanitarian crisis and infectious disease"-- Provided by publisher.
Identifiers: LCCN 2020052814 (print) | LCCN 2020052815 (ebook) | ISBN 9781509547791 (hardback) | ISBN 9781509547807 (paperback) | ISBN 9781509547814 (epub)
Subjects: LCSH: Epidemics--Political aspects. | Epidemiology--Political aspects.
Classification: LCC RA649 .D49 2021 (print) | LCC RA649 (ebook) | DDC 614.4--dc23
LC record available at https://lccn.loc.gov/2020052814
LC ebook record available at https://lccn.loc.gov/2020052815

Typeset in 10.75pt on 14pt Janson by
Servis Filmsetting Limited, Stockport, Cheshire
Printed and bound in Great Britain by TJ Books Ltd, Padstow, Cornwall

For further information on Polity, visit our website:
politybooks.com

Contents

Acknowledgements

This book began life as a compilation of reflections provisionally entitled 'Critical Thinking in a Pandemic', which became an essay in the 3 April 2020 online issue of *Boston Review*, entitled 'New Pathogen, Old Politics' (http://bostonreview.net/science-nature/alex-de-waal-new-pathogen-old-politics). The *Boston Review* editors, Deb Chasman and Matt Lord, were indulgent, encouraging, and usefully critical. I have drawn on comments and critique from colleagues, students, and former students, including Lisa Avery, Bridget Conley, Sarah Detzner, Ella Duncan, Sulmaan Khan, Jared Miller, Aditya Sarkar, and Ben Spatz, as well as Louise Knight and Inès Boxman at Polity Press and anonymous reviewers.

1

Following the Science, Following the Script

A pandemic pathogen is scary and strange. It is new to medical science and society and it is everywhere. At the critical early moment of a pandemic, much of the advice of doctors and epidemiologists will be vague and some will be wrong. Those who know their subject best will have the deepest uncertainties. No expert can say when and how the pandemic will end. There isn't even an agreed definition of 'pandemic' – an arcane but revealing absence.

Public leaders pay homage to 'following the science' but they actually follow a script. It's a storyline with a reassuring ending. It goes something like this:

> *We are at war against an invisible enemy. While our doctors and nurses combat the disease at the frontline in hospitals, while our scientists seek the cures and vaccines in their laboratories, the population must make sacrifices on the home front. We should trust our government while we forgo liberties and livelihoods. The pandemic will end with a medical magic bullet that vanquishes the pathogen. Then we will return to our way of life and be safe.*

This is the basic outline of a war story. It's also a tale of conquest of the microbial world and a charter for emergency rule that sets aside human rights and civil liberties. 'War on disease' is not a harmless metaphor. It suppresses critical thinking. It focuses our worries on a singular germ as our enemy, forgetting about other things – such as devastated ecologies and an inequitable society – that are no less pathogenic. And its comforting ending is false – even if the discovery of a vaccine or therapy means that leaders feel entitled to declare 'victory'.

This book is about this gargantuan and harmful error. It is about how and why the 'war on disease' script was written and how it guides our thinking and shapes our institutions in ways that we may not realize. When we most need a narrative to make sense of a devastating pandemic, the 'war on disease' not only fails, but also stops us recognizing our failures. This book is also about some very different visions. Scientists, social activists, and public health experts have other analyses and narratives – rigorous, practical, democratic, holistic – that we should pursue. The Covid-19 pandemic and crisis is showing us that the 'war on disease' is at best humdrum and at worst dangerous, and that these alternatives are urgent.

The 'war on disease' script is like the sheaf of documents in a desk drawer seldom opened. It consists of a handful of different scripts, pictures, and reminders. Some are Chinese, most are European or American. Also in the drawer are other images for disease outbreaks: a journey, an imbalance in the cosmos, a crime investigation, a storm, and a forest fire.[1]

In an emergency, we think fast and intuitively. To change the metaphor, being caught by a pandemic is like being caught in a storm when hiking in the mountains: suddenly the clouds roll in, darkness descends, rain lashes down, and the stones become slippery. We can't stay where we are, and we can't wait for the storm to clear to look around and find the best way down – we want to find a way to safety right away. There's a handrail: we grasp onto it because it keeps us steady. This handrail is our intuition, built from metaphors, storylines, images, and memories of what worked in the past. It's more than just a thesaurus, it's actually *how we think* – and so it usually goes unexamined. In the moment of greatest turmoil, fear, and uncertainty, it's reassuring. The handrail makes each step feel safe, and we assure ourselves that we can look at the map later on. That map will show us some other directions we might have taken, had we stopped to orient ourselves more carefully. We may regret that we didn't pause for a few moments to consider those other paths.

Following the Science

Experts on pandemics like the storm metaphor. The influential health scientist Michael Osterholm has compared an influenza pandemic to a blizzard and coronavirus to a hurricane.[2] In 2007, the United States Federal Government published a preparedness plan that adapted the five-level tropical storm classification scale for use in responding to epidemics (where a 'category 5' is the most destructive).[3] It grades national-level disease outbreaks in terms of fatalities. According to its rankings, Covid-19 in 2020 would be category 2 (that is, an order of magnitude less severe than some of the diseases anticipated.) The scale may be a useful prop for getting politicians to take notice, but it reproduces an elementary mistake. A pandemic isn't just a disease outbreak or epidemic multiplied to pan-continental size. Scale is important, for sure, but there's a qualitative aspect as well. The World Health Organization (WHO) stirred controversy in 2009 when it quietly changed its definition of an influenza pandemic. The previous definition was 'when a new influenza virus appears against which the human population has no immunity, resulting in several simultaneous epidemics worldwide with enormous numbers of deaths and illness'. The revised one cut out the words 'enormous numbers of deaths and illness'.[4] A pandemic that doesn't cause massive human suffering might seem odd to the layperson, but the virologists' particular concern is the *newness* of the pathogen and not how many people it sickens and kills. The novel coronavirus that causes Covid-19 is exactly such a candidate. Its closest relative is severe acute respiratory syndrome (SARS), which emerged in 2002, and it has some epidemiological similarities to influenza, but Covid-19 possesses characteristics all of its own.

For doctors, microbiologists, and epidemiologists, what matters in the storm isn't so much the wind but the darkness: we can't see our way. There's a trope among crisis epidemiologists: if you've seen one pandemic, you've seen just one pandemic.[5] The health metrics expert Chris Murray described constructing his model for Covid-19 as 'forecasting the weather while trying to build the forecasting tools'.[6] Perhaps we should adapt the storm metaphor to capture the fact that each pandemic isn't just a hurricane, it's a *new kind* of weather condition. Margaret Chan, Director General of the WHO in 2009, observed 'the virus writes the rules'.[7] Those rules govern how the disease is transmitted, which people are symptomatic and which are contagious and when, and what the microbe does to the human body and brain. It can take years to figure them out. In the case of the novel coronavirus, science has moved with unprecedented speed, but it is still lagging behind the epidemic curve. What we do during that lag is what's most important.

We like to think that biomedical scientists can provide authoritative certainty. As a pandemic hits, that isn't so. They are confident that their research methods will provide answers, but they don't have them yet. A new pathogen is an off-model event and models don't (by definition) predict them. In these events, it's the narrative that counts.[8] Scientists also have difficulty in explaining what their uncertainties mean to the public. In turn, every doubt or debate feeds the appetite of denialists, conspiracists, and pseudo-scientists, such as anti-vaxxers. In America, changes in advice to the public from the Centers for Disease Control and Prevention (CDC) in the early days of Covid-19 – initially advising against stopping incoming travellers from Europe and China[9] – have been repeatedly brought up by far-right pundits purportedly to show that public health authorities can't be trusted. Public health spokespeople and science journalists find that debating denialists registers somewhere between irritation and enraged despair. The difficulty is that the history of medicine includes enough moral outrages, good-faith errors, and unanticipated calamities to justify critical questioning. But leveraging these concerns to assail the whole edifice is to misunderstand the nature of scientific authority. To the religious dogmatist, authority is flat: all statements of scripture possess the same sacred quality, and to doubt one is to doubt all. To the scientific mind, theories are open to revision, technologies are not infallible, but facts are real.

Science is itself a journey. Every time the climbers reach a summit, they see a new vista of peaks and valleys to explore. The history of science shows that understanding a pandemic pathogen isn't merely an increment to existing medical knowledge but can also be a paradigm-shifting breakthrough. For each of the main pathogens examined in this book – cholera, influenza, and HIV, plus yellow fever and Ebola, which are covered more briefly – the search for prevention and cure has taken scientists into new terrain they could not have anticipated. Of all the sciences, medicine is the one most focused on the human being as such, and it is notable that it has been biologists who have blurred the boundaries of the human self, imputed agency to microbes, and in other ways challenged the distinction between the natural world and the human, so foundational to our modernist worldviews. Bruno Latour has made the same observation with regard to those hardest of hard scientists, geologists, who coined the word 'Anthropocene' to refer to our current era in which human activities are determining the global ecosystem. He writes: 'No postmodern philosopher, no anthropologist, no liberal theologian, no political thinker would have dared measure the influence of humans on the same scale as rivers, volcanos, erosion and biochemistry.'[10] In medicine as in geology, such critique doesn't come from post-modernist literary theorists, but from the Sherpas of scientific exploration themselves. We will see that this is the case for Covid-19 too.

A Week Is a Long Time

Pandemics move faster than politics. In the early acute phase, the number of cases of a disease can double every few days. It's a frightening trajectory. A week is a long time for a pathogen, as it is in politics.

Public leaders must act very quickly. Individuals who hold high office are, in general, attuned to their constituents' anxieties and what those may mean for the political order and their own political standing. They're not usually very literate in the science of infectious diseases and they don't have time to learn anything new and complicated. At that moment of darkness and uncertainty as the pandemic storm breaks, ministers and presidents want reassurance – for themselves and so they can provide leadership in the hour of crisis. Their task is to control the narrative, to buy time and calm, so that public health and medicine can control the disease.

A government leader has scientific advisers. For medical issues, that means biomedical scientists. The hierarchy of academic disciplines becomes desperately important at this moment of crisis because this is the order in which the decision-maker consults them, and the weight that their advice carries. This is shown by Nancy Krieger, who compares the number of projects funded by the US National Institutes of Health for the hard biomedical sciences as against social epidemiology: the ratio is 25 to one. Peer-reviewed publications favour the hard biomedical sciences 194 to one.[11] Between the academic top table and the rest of the scholarly hall there's a huge step down – more of a precipice than a gradient. Next in the ranking are the epidemiological modellers, below them the social epidemiologists, and last the medical anthropologists and historians. Ecological scientists sit somewhere in the middle. This hierarchy corresponds roughly to the 'hardness' of the science, and depending on where a researcher sits, everyone above him or her is a true 'hard scientist' and everyone below a 'soft' one. It's a gendered hierarchy – there are far fewer women in the higher reaches. Those at the farthest end of the hall – who study literature, history, and social anthropology – like to critique and deconstruct the hierarchy and mock the pretensions of those at the top. Meanwhile, hard scientists tend to go soft-headed when they cross the boundary into social and political analysis – they turn to platitude and metaphor. They know what *ought* to be done: it's just a matter for the public, or society, or whoever, to get on and do it.

Most scientists' approach to public messaging has been that facts speak for themselves. This hasn't worked. Towards the end of his book *Spillover*, the journalist David Quammen inadvertently shows how scientific thinking loses its compass as it crosses this divide. In 500 pages, he vividly describes the work of virologists who hunt down and analyse pathogens that have either made the zoonotic jump from animals to humans or have a fearsome potential do so. It's fascinating. These scientists are, he says, 'our sentries' who will 'raise the alarm'. Quammen continues: 'What happens after that will depend upon science, politics, and social mores, public opinion, public will, and other forms of human behavior. It depends on how we citizens respond.' Those ways of responding are 'either calmly or hysterically, either intelligently or doltishly'.[12] This is true but it also doesn't get us far: social scientists and political analysts have useful things to say on these topics. They too have their hierarchy, with economists at the top table. But a pandemic is a rare occasion in which economists don't have a model to hand,[13] though they have much to say about what can be done to mitigate the crises of paying for health care, unemployment, and disruption to international trade. Macroeconomic models that take equilibrium as a premise don't work when – as in a pandemic – there is by definition no equilibrium.

Politicians talk to their friends and financiers in business, who are also used to making complex decisions quickly in uncertain situations. Business school methods that focus on real-world problems can be useful when the data are speculative and the quantitative formulae have just been thrown out of the window. The core business management question is 'what is going on here?' and the answer is given by means of a story that makes sense. So far so good. That works when our intuitions have been refined by experiences that fit the problem. But it doesn't work when the problem follows a new logic for which our thinking need to be rewired – for example a novel pathogen.

The security advisers have a narrative too. Their job includes planning for a full spectrum of hazards, including all manner of nasty surprises. Military officers and intelligence analysts have played out wargames with both humans and natural disasters as the enemy 'red team' and have watched how decision-makers respond to the stresses of the unexpected. One of those exercises, repeated every year or so in governments of industrialized countries, is the crisis of a highly contagious germ introduced either by a terrorist with access to a high-security biotech laboratory, or by natural spillover. So the security analysts consider themselves ready – or at least a step ahead of others. But they can't anticipate what rules a new virus might follow. They also suffer the handicap of those tasked with imagining the unanticipated, which is that in order to make their story credible – plausible enough to convince a jaded politician – they can only break one or two rules about normality at a time. In the same way that a science fiction movie stretches our imagination on one dimension but sticks to a conventional plotline and characterization so as not to bewilder the audience, so too the pandemic disaster scenario hews to an intuitively resonant human script. These rules are written by the scriptwriter. This is why, almost inevitably, the reality of a pandemic will be stranger than fiction or a security studies wargame simulation. This naturally won't become clear until later. In emergency mode – and most politicians have an adrenaline rush when there is a real emergency, with top-secret briefings with the highest-ranking generals and spy chiefs – those security-based narratives, scary but familiar, will resonate.

Routinely, a political leader will talk to other politicians. The normal calculus of day-to-day politicking about loyalty, jobs, money, and the media doesn't stop. We hope that in a national emergency, all those become secondary to the public good. One of the virtues of a pandemic-as-national-security drama is that it allows a leader to rise above party politics and set a truly national agenda, even a global one. Every politician also knows that they should never let a crisis go to waste. For some, the chance for partisan gain trumps the public good. There are benefits to pandemics: an opportunity to seize emergency powers and use them to other ends, spend public money with little oversight, and get on with other factional business while public attention is distracted. Some leaders are denialists. A few are devout denialists, who genuinely think the disease is a hoax or truly have faith that religious piety is sufficient to prevail. Others are tactical denialists, for whom challenging the science or letting turmoil spread brings immediate political advantages. More common are those who pay enough attention to half-convince themselves of a simplified storyline, and then screen out contradictory information.

In a crisis, political leaders don't usually consult the people, because it's complicated and takes time and they don't know what questions to pose. For those who are genuinely committed to democracy, or to finding the best all-of-society way through the crisis, it's a short-cut that they will come to regret. But the mistake is easily made because there's no readily available template for a democratic pandemic response.

The 'War on Disease' Storyline

It should be clear by now that science cannot provide certainty for political decisions in the moment of a fast-moving pandemic. The 'war on disease' storyline steps in for that purpose. The reason why government leaders find it useful is because it's reassuring. Unfortunately its reassurances are false. To call on a new metaphor, the warfighting script is like those well-worn, half-forgotten clothes at the back of the wardrobe that are pulled out for an unexpected occasion. They don't really fit but there's nothing else to wear on the day. And besides, they are at least inconspicuous because everyone else is wearing something similar. Hence the title of this book: the pathogen is novel and unpredictable, the political scripts are familiar and predictable from the first word to the last.

We shouldn't take the martial language too literally, and those who know it are well aware that it's not a 'real' war. Scientists and public health experts see it as a way of validating their work, as an innocent cover story that appeals to a spirit of solidarity and selflessness and helps us cope with dangers and setbacks. Those are fair considerations, but the script has other consequences too. Policies are standardized and imposed by decree. The archetype is how the German imperial government defeated cholera in Hamburg, described at the end of chapter 2, and the American army's conquest of yellow fever in Cuba, Panama, and the southern United States, described at the beginning of chapter 3. The way in which HIV and AIDS policies became part of an international security regime is examined in chapter 4, and in chapter 5 I will show some of the errors made by militarizing the response to Ebola. In America, the role of soldiers in 'fighting' diseases helps validate the apparently limitless expansion of the tasks given to the Pentagon – a definitional inflation that makes 'war' at once all-encompassing and meaningless.

Declaring war is also declaring a state of emergency, which is a temptation to autocrats. Labelling the microbe as an 'invisible enemy' or an 'invader' can imply that those who carry it are also enemies or invaders. In America, the term 'lockdown', innocuous in the white suburbs, has the resonance of the New Jim Crow among communities familiar with mass incarceration, where locking down prisoners in their cells is the routine response to a prison disturbance. Lockdowns may provide some immediate safety from physical injury to prisoners but their intent is to protect the prison itself. In countries familiar with civil war and counter-insurgency, the rhetoric and physical attributes of lockdown, such as checkpoints, curfews, and neighbourhood searches, are reminders that there is a thin line between policing a pathogen and policing a hostile population. The warlike language means that advocates for democracy, equity, and justice are constantly at a disadvantage, as their dissent may be seen as sabotaging the war effort.

The 'war on disease' is also a script for conquest. The European version was born exactly at the zenith of colonial ambition and still carries that imperial DNA, as a project for dominion over the territories of the globe, its peoples and its microbes. Its language is male, white, and controlling. It promises mastery over nature, setting our bounds wider still and wider, making our mighty technologies mightier yet. This is perhaps its most insidious implication: a victory over a disease is a validation of a benevolent (for us) Anthropocene.

Fighting words also serve politicians whose agenda is dominating the day's headlines. In the last few years, legal-rational forms of public authority have yielded to charismatic, transactional, and disruptive styles of governing. For such politicians, the narrative *is* the solution, and science should be strictly in its service. Donald Trump was an exemplar. Transactional politicians such as he are tactical fighters, not strategic war planners. They relish political combat but don't want the institutional discipline of organizing a war effort, and choose their fighting talk accordingly. Like others who deny or disregard scientific method and data, Trump did so against a background of unquestioned faith in other things – in his case, winning through acts of will and rhetoric. And while he considered face masks and restrictions on travelling and congregating as something between an annoyance and a conspiracy, he believed fervently in the catechism of the magic bullet, perhaps even more so than his scientifically literate political peers.

The main topic of this book is the construction and reconstruction of the Euro-American 'war on disease' narrative. I chose three historical pandemics for this purpose. Cholera is the case in chapter 2. This is where Europe's war on disease began two hundred years ago, as a handful of metaphors, images, and practices. Of these the most consequential was the concept of policing the contagious, inherited from the plague and applied to cholera. At that time, the idea of a 'war' that resembled a real war would have been fanciful. That changed, and by the end of the 19th century a firm storyline took shape. Its first element was the plan of campaign – an assemblage of instruments for social control, which we could distil into a slogan: lookout, cleanup, and lockdown. 'Lookout' was alertness for cases, especially sick travellers, and detecting the pathways of disease spread. 'Cleanup' was sanitation: personal cleanliness, fresh air, clean drinking water, draining stagnant water in which insects might breed, controlling vermin and disposing of sewage and rubbish. 'Lockdown' was quarantine, sequestration, isolation, and curfew – policing people and pathogens. The next operation in the war story was conquest and dominion: the project of exploring, naming, classifying, and controlling the entire surface of the planet and every living thing upon it, from microbes to human beings to forests. In short: imperial exploration, expansion, and subjugation. The final element was the technology for victory, when microbiologists began crafting 'magic bullets' that could hit those invisible enemies.

Chapter 3 deals with influenza in 1918–19: a pandemic that refuted civilization's proudest achievements. It was a monstrous killer and, insofar as there was a fight against it, influenza won. The Great War created and transmitted the virus, public health measures worked only at the margin, and medical science found neither cure nor vaccine. But the script served its purposes: governments continued to mobilize armies and send them to the warfront and citizens kept faith in biomedicine. The failure and deceit over influenza were too big to contemplate, and the pandemic remained untold history for two generations. Virulent influenza was our social taboo, but our virological totem: fear of its return energized pandemic preparedness in the 21st century.

The war on disease was refashioned after World War II, when international health campaigns against smallpox and polio registered huge gains. The successes were such that the medical academy was ready to declare victory over infectious diseases altogether. This was hubris. In chapter 4, I turn to a momentous setback with a surprising twist: HIV/AIDS. The story of the global response to this pandemic is inspiring – and also confounds the standard narrative. A coalition of people living with HIV/AIDS and a wider community of carers, physicians, and global health advocates pursued an agenda of health and human rights, which surpassed expectations on both counts. They sometimes used fighting language, but in the different sense of a struggle for liberation and emancipation. AIDS was exceptional, however. For other 'emerging and re-emerging' infectious diseases, the 'war on disease' was reinvented. This is the focus of chapter 5. After the millennium, fears of unknown or resurgent pathogens that threatened 'Pandemic X' re-militarized pandemic preparedness. Advocates for global health security found a storyline in common with the war on terror. Our fears and efforts were targeted on individual germs, and not on the ecologies that generate them or the society and economy that enable them to spread.

The history of the 'war on disease' narrative is an ironic commentary on medicine and warmaking. Microbes have decided the outcome of wars, though generals on the winning side don't often acknowledge it. Military doctors have been leaders in the technologies of controlling contagious diseases, and their medical victories have enabled armies to complete conventional forms of conquest, such as expanding empires. Military scientists have also created monstrous bio-weapons in the laboratory. Pandemic preparedness intersects with biosecurity risks when a laboratory engineers a virulent pathogen to discover more about the pandemic threats we may face, with the aim of better understanding and counteracting them. A pathogen like this may escape through a laboratory accident (which has happened a number of times, though scientists prefer not to talk about it, as described in chapter 5), and once an academic journal has published the genetic codes for a virulent virus, it's possible for a malevolent scientist to repeat the feat.

Covid-19 was the least unexpected pandemic in history. Scientific and institutional preparations narrowed the uncertainties of a new pathogen to a span that should have been readily manageable. And indeed the development of vaccines in record time is testament to scientific expertise backed by public money. The best-laid plans were confounded, however. It turned out that the main agent of radical uncertainty was not a new and inscrutable microbe. Instead it was Anglo-American political leaders whose doctrine of disrupting institutions, including science, made the pandemic ungovernable. At a cost of hundreds of thousands of dead and millions impoverished, this has had the modest virtue of showing that the 'war on disease' is a humdrum script that cannot guide political action.

Towards Democratic, Ecological Public Health

I would have liked to have drafted a new playbook for emancipatory public health in the Anthropocene, but this book concludes with something more modest: an appeal that it's necessary to talk about this. There are hopeful openings, such as 'One Health', which unifies public health with animal health and environmental sustainability, and 'people's science' approaches to disease control. At the moment, however, these remain minority agendas.

For now, people who work for democracy, human rights, liberal education, environmental sustainability, and similar goals – citizens, activists, elected officials, and the like – are bewildered as a pandemic arrives. They shouldn't be. For English-speakers at least, their problem begins because the English language doesn't give them a firm mental grip on the crisis. Our vocabulary is deficient.

The point of etymological origin is the word 'epidemic'. This was first used by Hippocrates 2,500 years ago. In classical Athens, an 'epidemic' referred to an episode of sicknesses among the people. The people ('*demos*') was not today's 'population', it was restricted to free male citizens. Sicknesses included all diseases occurring at the time. In the 14th century, 'epidemic' got attached to named diseases, especially plague. Often used interchangeably with the noun 'epidemy', in the early 19th century, 'pandemic' was used for a geographically magnified epidemic. Cholera was its archetype. At first, it had a sibling 'pandemy' as well. With the demise of 'epidemy' and 'pandemy', the English language lost the distinction between a societal crisis and a much higher number of cases than normal of a disease.[14] 'Pandemic' is best used as an adjective, to qualify a disease – thus, 'pandemic influenza' or 'pandemic Covid-19'. Were these old words to be revived, speaking of the 'Covid-19 pandemy' would make it clear that we're referring to the entire societal crisis. This crisis includes all the other health problems that worsen when hospitals are overwhelmed by cases of one disease, along with the psychological distress, the losses of livelihoods, and strains on communities. The concept 'pandemy' could also be stretched to include ecological and societal pathologies that cause pandemics. I won't use the word 'pandemy' in the chapters that follow, but it will remain in the background and I will return to it in the final chapter.

Democrats and social activists don't have many tools to steady them in the pandemic storm. They can look to historians' accounts of past pandemies (here the word doesn't sound so quaint), but each one of those is so distinct, and the context in which they struck is so different, that there doesn't appear to be much of current relevance. Reading Boccaccio on the plague in Italy, or Daniel Defoe's account of the London plague, or reconstructing the devastations of small-pox in 16th-century Mexico, provides a stock of anecdotes and intriguing echoes but not much more. This book is also a history, but my guiding principle is that each pandemic is a shock and disruption of its own distinct kind. Insofar as there's a pattern, it's in the political response.

We can turn to social medicine and its analysis of inequal-ities in health care provision and health outcomes, and the importance of socially engaged and culturally sensitive public health.[15] Each pandemic reveals inequalities in health, hous-ing, income, and political access. HIV/AIDS shone a light on other injustices: discrimination, stigma, sexual and gen-der-based violence and exploitation, and repressive policing. With Covid-19, selective vaccine provision may soon become the greatest ever inequality in health care history. Social medicine also illuminates the frightening levels of public dis-trust in medical expertise. For too long, health experts and authorities took public compliance for granted. Today, 'trust me, I'm a doctor' no longer convinces. Minorities and for-merly colonized peoples have had good reasons to distrust the official health apparatus, which too often treated them with contempt. Western publics are growing suspicious of medical authorities, to the extent that mass vaccination – the single greatest success of public health – is in serious peril. Vaccination prevents epidemics when it delivers herd immu-nity, which is usually achieved when about two-thirds of the population have natural or acquired immunity. Vaccine dis-trust means that America and some other countries may not be able to reach that threshold for Covid-19. Most health scientists just want these problems to go away: the facts alone should suffice to convince. In her book on this subject, *Stuck*, Heidi Larson takes a different view. She provoca-tively observes that 'vaccine rumors are here to stay, but that is not a bad thing'.[16] That's because medical scientists are compelled to join the public debate – a debate that will need to include questioning the role of immunological technology in the Anthropocene. Expedited comprehensive immunization is akin to building higher seawalls to protect coasts from the rising oceans: inescapable but limited.

The citizen science movement has been hugely accelerated by Covid-19. Never before have so many people become epidemiologically numerate so quickly. But this hasn't kept pace with a fast-raging pandemic. The most encouraging examples of activists setting an agenda for pandemic response are from HIV/AIDS – which I will discuss in chapter 4 – but that was a slow-burn pandemic and it took several years for the affected communities to organize and make their case, and for the health authorities to listen. In the case of Ebola in west Africa – discussed in chapter 5 – the mutual learning was much quicker and the anthropologist Paul Richards observes that the epidemic was overcome when 'communities learnt to think like epidemiologists, and epidemiologists to think like communities'.[17] This is a crucial example of public health as a people's science, and Richards encouragingly observes that it can happen rapidly.

Joint learning by epidemiologists and the public runs into several problems with the 'war on disease'. The first is that war leaders give orders and expect obedience.

The second is that control instruments demand discipline. For contagious diseases, it's a brute fact that measures such as stopping travel and screening or quarantining travellers, and rigorous surveillance of individuals' activities, *can* stop transmission. In European history, building and legitimizing that apparatus of control was part of creating the state.[18] Human rights law allows for emergency public health to overrule civil and political rights.[19] The tensions between disease containment and personal freedoms are real, but are easily exaggerated and politicized, especially when narratives of control and fear chime with authoritarianism and xenophobia. Measures to control infectious diseases don't need to be coercive and comprehensive. The opposite is true: they work best when they are consensual and precise – the two go together because contagion control is best done locally by ordinary people. The most encouraging examples of joint learning by communities and epidemiologists are in the global south or among minorities.

This points to a third problem with the 'war on disease': its imperial lineage. Rich countries typically don't have the humility to accept lessons from former colonies. An African slave introduced smallpox inoculation to North America in 1720 but his contribution isn't widely known and his real name isn't known at all. Recent Ebola outbreaks were overcome by African people's science, and one of the saddest episodes in Covid-19 policy is that African countries have not valued that experience and have instead regressed to copying centrally planned European lockdowns, which are hopelessly ill suited to their circumstances. Again, we can also learn from AIDS. Many of the most effective HIV prevention programmes were set up in partnership with injecting drug users and sex workers. We would all be much safer if we could respect 'the wisdom of whores'.[20]

Social activists and social scientists are unprepared for pandemics. They don't even have a paradigm to shift. What they do – consult, reflect, discuss – seems like a leisurely enterprise suited to a less urgent time, that is, afterwards. Implicitly, we accept centrally directed, expert-designed, and coercive measures because we assume they are a stopgap until biomedicine delivers a definitive cure. The technical term for behavioural and social measures is 'non-pharmaceutical interventions', or NPIs – which betrays their second-level standing. But these NPIs *are* the response, and because they are necessary and painful, it is important to have public discussion and consent. Can this be done fast? A year after Covid-19 appeared, it's evident that it should have been done at the beginning.

Those who believe they have 'won' a war are least likely to appraise candidly why they have prevailed, crediting successes to their skill and perseverance and not to their enemies' blunders – and still less to extraneous factors such as that under-appreciated arbiter of the battlefield, disease. Winners can be slow learners. This book also shows how historic 'victories' in the 'war on disease' have led to hubris or amnesia. Biomedical advances such as vaccines deliver genuine public goods, but – as virologists today appreciate – that is no cause for complacency. Which brings us to our last and biggest challenge.

The 'war on disease' also doesn't speak about the ravages of ecological destruction and the resulting disaster for the health of living things, including us. It makes microbes into enemies to be eliminated. Our conquest and dominion over the planet are on course to be the ultimate Pyrrhic victory. This is the calamitous Anthropocene: the result not of people as such, but of the organization of resource exploitation, manufacturing and agro-industrial production, massively concentrated human habitation and accentuated movement. Ecologists have been warning that deforestation and loss of wetlands are disrupting the habitats of bats, monkeys, and wild geese, risking more and more viral spillovers, and that industrial farming and urbanization are creating dangerous ecologies where viruses adapt more rapidly. Doctors have also been warning about the fast-approaching post-antibiotic era brought about by the reckless overuse of antibiotics, both by over-prescription by physicians and pharmacies, and in industrial livestock and fish farming. The new global ecology has been created by us but microbes are the quickest to adapt to it. The political-economic logics at work here are similar to those driving global heating and the climate crisis: the political clout, money, and readiness to lie and cheat by the corporations that profit from over-exploiting the planet are more powerful than the counter-pressure for responsible stewardship. Today, medical scientists and epidemiologists are joining environmental scientists in insisting that it isn't enough to identify and eliminate the next microbial culprits for contagious disease: we have also to stop the ecological devastation that is generating them. Each pandemic pathogen has forced science to think more deeply about the nature of disease. So too it compels us to think differently about how society is organized and politics is run. Pandemic Covid-19, along with its causes and social crises, is a chance for the urgent and inescapable task of rethinking *Homo sapiens'* place on this planet that we have too long considered ours.

2

The Rage of Numbers: Cholera

Robert Koch was one of the most eminent scientists of his age. He won a cabinet of awards, including a Nobel Prize for his discovery of the pathogen causing tuberculosis. At the end of his career, he reflected, 'My favourite decoration is my Imperial Crown Medal II Class, which our old Emperor personally bestowed on me after we returned from the cholera campaign to India. It is to be worn on a black-and-white ribbon, like a military decoration. And that is exactly what it was.'[1]

Koch had isolated the bacillus responsible for cholera in February 1884 in Calcutta and three months later returned to Berlin as a hero. He was elevated to the Privy Council and made de facto commander of all efforts to protect the empire from communicable diseases. Kaiser Wilhelm I, 87 years old at the time, compared the victory over cholera to Germany's defeat of France in 1870. Waging 'war' on an epidemic disease was an unlikely idea, but in the 1880s it began to take hold in the popular imagination. Koch's triumph was not only as a scientist, but also as political scriptwriter.

It's worth reflecting just how unexpected the story of 'war on disease' would have appeared at the time.

Kaiser Wilhelm and his senior military officers will have recalled the cholera pandemic of 1831, which had claimed the lives of Field Marshal General August von Gneisenau and his chief of staff, General Carl von Clausewitz. Not only did the disease kill two eminent soldiers, but their final military operation had been the enforcement of a cordon sanitaire intended to keep cholera out of Germany. It failed: cholera ravaged Berlin and then reached Paris, London, and other European cities the following year. After his death, Clausewitz became the most influential military theorist of the century. *On War* (*Vom Kriege*)[2] is regarded as the definitive account of all aspects of war. But it scarcely mentions disease. Clausewitz would have regarded his last command as a disagreeable police operation, not a war.

Throughout history, wars have been agents of fever and infectious diseases have been camp followers. The average soldier was more likely to be fodder for cholera than cannon; more died from bacilli than bullets. Courtiers, doctors, soldiers, and merchants might talk casually about cholera being an 'invader' or 'attacker' but that did not go further than a figure of speech. Outbreaks of disease were seen chiefly as a product of merciless and inscrutable nature, possibly foreseeable, like eclipses, certainly uncontrollable, like earthquakes or hailstorms. Epidemics shaped history but could not themselves be shaped; no sensible lessons could be drawn from their visitations. Thucydides, in the *History of the Peloponnesian War*, recounted the plague that ravaged Athens at the time of its defeat, but generations of staff college instructors used this classic text to illuminate strategy, making only passing mention of the calamitous epidemic. Since the medieval plagues, city authorities had attended to how they might *police* disease – or, more precisely, the people they suspected to be bearers of disease – but any soldiers dispatched to enforce plague regulations were not soldiering. War, instead, was a contest among princes resolved by valour, strength, and good fortune – or it was mayhem. Thomas Hobbes wrote of 'warre' as a condition of anarchy, hunger, and poverty. He used similes drawn from popular medicine to describe the ills that 'warre' afflicted on the body politic, but not the converse. To 'fight' a real disease made no more sense than 'fighting' against bad weather.

This changed in the half-century between Clausewitz's death and Koch's triumph, when the modern German state was built in the image of its army. To expand on Charles Tilly's phrase, while war made the state and the state made war, infectious disease was the arbiter of both.[3] The logic of microbial transmission imposed a new rigour on the regulation of international trade, the design of European cities, and the organization of war. The triangle of state, war, and medicine was knitted together by a new popular narrative about epidemic disease control, carved against the grain of centuries of experience: medicine became war-fighting. It was an odd and untheorized analogy but nonetheless took hold in a powerful way. The first imagined referent for 'war on disease' was imperial conquest.

Cholera as Protagonist

A century after Clausewitz, a Harvard immunologist wrote the first history that properly acknowledged pathogens' leading role in war. Hans Zinsser had served as a sanitary inspector for the US army in 1918 and had been offended by the demeaning way in which generals treated the junior officers assigned to protect their troops from infectious diseases. In his book *Rats, Lice and History*, he cut his superiors down to size. Zinsser awarded his medal to typhus, the louse-borne fever that was the long-standing fellow-traveller of armies, especially in cold climes, because the lice thrive in blankets and unwashed clothes, but cholera gets a mention in dispatches:

Soldiers have rarely won wars. They more often mop up after the barrage of epidemics. And typhus, with its brothers and sisters – plague, cholera, typhoid, dysentery – has decided more campaigns than Caesar, Hannibal, Napoleon, and the inspectors general of history. The epidemics get the blame for defeat, the generals get the credit for victory. It ought to be the other way around.[4]

Zinsser develops his theme and presents typhus as a character deserving a historical biography in its own right. He portrays the bacterium *Rickettsia prowazekii* as a relentless and resilient individual with a life story that spans centuries.[5] Geddes Smith, who wrote an popular introduction to epidemiology a few years later, used a different plotline: pathogens as hidden culprits for crimes, and the epidemiologist as detective set on solving a murder mystery.[6] A microbe *is* an agent, but it does not possess inner life, let alone motive. Its actions are ruled solely by the laws of natural selection. However, anthropomorphizing the microbes serves two purposes. First, it helps tell a story, and evolution has bestowed different bacteria and viruses with traits that can be portrayed like personalities. And second, it is important for human beings to explore the agency of other species and lifeforms – especially as so much of our own bodies consists of bacteria, and so much of our genome is the remnants of viral DNA.[7]

If we were to personify the cholera bacillus, it would be as a pantomime villain: naïve, gross, and savage. In later chapters, we will encounter other pathogenic protagonists which have more complicated personalities. Cholera is a simpleton chancer that tries its luck with humans as if it were playing a slot machine, winning a few coins here and there which it stuffs back into the slot for another try, until it strikes it lucky by getting its host to disgorge so many coins that the trays overflow. Once in the human body, a single cholera bacillus has something like a one in a million chance of prospering in the human gut. It must survive the stomach acid and it has to compete with the existing biota. But if it manages to lodge in the lining of the small intestine, the unimpeded progression of cholera bacillus runs something like this. It releases a toxin that causes the intestinal cells to release a torrent of water, which washes out its competitors and allows it to reproduce at a prodigious rate, making a copy of itself every 13 minutes. A single replicating bacillus, starting in the early morning, could in principle generate a population of over 8 billion copies by lunchtime – enough to cause acute symptoms. By the evening, that would be 8 billion squared – a savage arithmetic indeed. What that level of infection means for the affected person is, first, uncontrollable diarrhoea and vomiting. The body disgorges fluids, and it is this massive dehydration and loss of essential salts that can be lethal.[8] Today, at the first sign of the disease, a health worker provides oral rehydration therapy: water, sugar, and salt taken by mouth – a ridiculously simple treatment that is very effective. A grievously sick patient can then be hooked up to an intravenous feed. Two hundred years ago, people simply didn't know what to do except mop up what they called the 'dejecta' and pray. As the symptoms worsen, the person begins to turn blue and lose control of his or her nervous system, leading to spasms which may continue even after death.

The common name of the disease has an appropriately simple etymology: the Greek *kholera*, the Latin *cholera*, and the Middle English *choler* all mean diarrhoea. In Galenic medicine, *choler* branched out to also mean bile or anger, one of the four bodily humours: phlegmatic, choleric, sanguine, and melancholic; disease was supposed to occur when these were out of balance. Its scientific name is also straightforward: the bacterium has the shape of a comma, which gives its movements something of a wriggle, and when Koch isolated it, he simply called it *Vibrio cholerae*. He claimed to have isolated *the* cause of the disease, and to have refuted rival scientists who had more complex explanations based on the peculiarities of the natural environment or the physiology of the individual patient.

The complete story of cholera is more complicated. Hundreds of variant forms of the comma bacillus are found among the rich bacterial life of warm-water estuaries around the world. They have no natural host, but readily attach themselves to the shells of crustaceans. Only two strains possess an additional section of chromosome that has the genes for secreting a toxin that changes the bacteria from being harmless to a killer of humans. This was presumably acquired during some random microbial encounter.[9] These toxic versions are endemic in the river deltas of Bengal. They can find their way to the human intestine when people eat undercooked shellfish, drink contaminated water, or eat fruit or vegetables that have been washed in such water. Most people who ingest the bacillus have only mild or symptomless infections. The fact that an asymptomatic person can be infectious, albeit slightly and for a short period, means that the pathogen can spread unnoticed, and therefore can travel silently for a distance. When the disease progresses, it does so very quickly: acute symptoms develop within a day, at most two. This is when the bacterium hits the jackpot whereupon billions of copies spill out in dejecta to be passed on. A sick person can infect his or her household members and carers, and anyone who comes into contact with fomites (contaminated inanimate objects) such as soiled clothing or bedding.[10] If that person's faeces spill into a well or river, the outbreak can spread further.

Cholera on the March

Indians were familiar with the toxic strain of cholera for centuries, as an endemic disease in the delta of the Ganges-Brahmaputra in Bengal with occasional epidemics up and down the coast, on occasion killing thousands of people.[11] These outbreaks were contained because people didn't move around fast enough. Cholera exhausted itself because the population of locally susceptible people would acquire immunity through infections (mostly mild or inapparent), or they would die. In the 1770s, when the East India Company seized control of Bengal, it brought with it ruthless exploitation and one of the worst famines in history. And in a kind of microbial revenge, cholera then travelled along the routes of conquest and export all the way back to Europe, ultimately reaching London. Doctors named it 'Asiatic cholera' to distinguish it from familiar diarrhoeal afflictions.

The first time that cholera travelled outside India was in 1817–21. We don't know whether the existing strain mutated to become more virulent or whether it was simply the existing pattern of local outbreaks magnified to imperial scale. But we do know that it was devastating. Drawing on the reports of James Jameson of the Bengal Medical Board, the historian David Arnold provides a vivid account of how it afflicted an army mobilized by the East India Company:

> After 'creeping about . . . in its unwonted insidious manner' for several days among the 'lower classes of the camp followers,' the disease suddenly, [Jameson] wrote, 'gained fresh vigour, and at once burst forth with irresistible violence in every direction.' In a short time there were so many casualties that the medical staff could not cope with them all.[12]

The commander, blaming the disease on the fact that they had pitched camp in an unhealthy spot, ordered the brigade to move. From his 11,500 soldiers, 764 died in a single week. Jameson writes about cholera as a kind of guerrilla assailing the army. It would be equally accurate to describe the army itself as the agent of infection. Arnold writes of 'the literal correspondence between cholera and military power in colonial India. . . . To speak of the "invasion" of cholera as if it were an army on the march was thus more than a casual analogy.'[13]

By sea, cholera sailed both east (reaching China) and west (to Mesopotamia). It was transported by ships, but whether this was through contagion or because of the foul miasmas that built up in cargo holds during voyages wasn't clear at the time. Either way, the pandemic coincided with the first shipments of cotton from India to Manchester factories. Its transmission was aided by merchants who were adamant that the price of cotton unloaded at the Liverpool docks wouldn't be competitive if the additional costs for 65 days' quarantine were added. They pressed parliament to pass a Quarantine Act in 1825 that simplified and reduced the disparate sanitary regulations and quarantine requirements.[14] Cholera also travelled by land through Afghanistan and Persia, and along the Russian military roads in the Caucasus mountains to reach southern Russia.

This first pandemic of Asiatic cholera faded away by 1823, but not for long. Just a few years later, a second pandemic followed much the same routes. The disease wasn't only terrifying but was confusing too. At times, it was clear that it closely followed the movement of people, but then it seemed to disappear for a while before erupting unexpectedly in a new place. We can now be sure that pilgrims and merchants travelling through the mountain passes carried cholera from the cities of the Indus valley to Afghanistan and Persia. Some of those carriers would have been asymptomatic. Contemporary writers 'generally assumed that it was blown over the tops of the Himalaya and Suleiman mountains'.[15] Cholera again followed trade routes to southern Russia, and in August 1830 reached the annual fair at Nishni Novgorod. There, traders congregated from Moscow and other Russian cities, as well as from Hungary, Austria, and Poland.

The merchants and the burghers of the Russian trading cities repeated the arguments heard in Manchester. The disease couldn't possibly be spread by human traffic – and therefore quarantining ships and sequestrating cities would be useless. They supported the 'miasma' view: it was a disease generated by local conditions and carried by the wind. Others took a third view: the disease was harboured in particular local conditions, probably the soil, waiting for an unknown element to cause it erupt.

During the previous pandemic, Tsar Nicholas I of Russia initially sided with medical advisers who said that cholera was a contagious disease.[16] In 1830, he vacillated, adopting an amalgam of all three prevalent theories: miasmatism, contagionism, and localism. (Confusingly for us, miasmatism was sometimes called infectionism, as it held that the disease was infectious through the air, as opposed to spread by direct contact.) But as reports arrived of cholera's advance towards Moscow, Nicholas ordered his army units to stop it, setting in train what the historian Charlotte Henze has called 'Europe's great experiment in eradicating cholera with anti-plague defences'.[17] In most of Europe, the plague-control handbook was an archive of practices from long before living memory, but in Russia the last visitation of the plague had been as recently as 1770, when it spread from the empire's southern marches as far as Moscow, causing a riot. Exclusionary methods of plague control suited autocrats, and Empress Catherine blamed the Tatars and sundry peoples of the eastern borderlands.

In 1830, as cholera approached, Tsar Nicholas ordered a double line of soldiers around Moscow with loaded cannons ready to fire on wagons or boats that breached the cordon. Army units dismantled small bridges and blocked big ones. They confiscated horses and carts. Anyone showing signs of sickness was isolated and their clothes were washed in chlorine water or fumigated, by soldiers who probably didn't have much idea of what they were doing.[18] But still cholera reached Moscow. At that time, the imperial capital was St Petersburg, and the tsar ordered a triple cordon of troops to surround the city and more units to enforce what we would now call a lockdown. That caused a riot. People were more outraged by the suppression of their livelihoods than the disease and blamed the authorities for poisoning them, and attacked doctors, officials, and foreigners.[19] The military policy was, as Henze writes, 'a complete failure'.[20]

Clausewitz and Cholera

In the first weeks of 1831, Carl von Clausewitz left his home at the military college in Breslau to take a new military assignment. He was chief of staff to the Prussian army's eastern forces on an operation to protect the kingdom against an invasion of Asiatic cholera. Though Clausewitz and his contemporaries never used the term, this mission has a good claim to be considered modern Europe's first 'war on disease'.

The Prussian King Frederick Wilhelm III assembled medical experts in an 'Immediate Commission' who studied everything they could discover about cholera and its control, including what English officials such as Dr Jameson had recently written and the Westminster parliamentary debates of 1825. They also reviewed the Habsburg imperial government's reactivation of medieval plague-control measures on its Balkan frontiers. They received a delegation from Paris, the capital of European medical science.

The first anti-plague handbook had been drafted in Italian and Adriatic city-states in the years after the apocalyptic shock of the 1348 Black Death. The plague arrived explosively and killed in a gruesome and rapid way. Its mortality rate was extraordinarily high: overall, perhaps a third of the population of Asia and Europe succumbed, and in most European cities, half of the residents perished, sometimes in just a few weeks. Then the plague came back after a few years, again and again over three centuries. Popular explanations attributed it to divine wrath, astronomical alignments, witchcraft, and sorcery. Italian princes, city elders, and merchants were more empirical.[21] The earliest boards of health were set up in Venice and Florence in the same year that the plague first appeared; these evolved into permanent magistracies over the next century, with authority to restrict travel and trade, and isolate infected individuals. Isolation hospitals, called *lazzaretti*, were set up to prevent contagion.

Italian cities also issued certificates of health to important traders and diplomats, so that they could pass freely through checkpoints. The first passports were health cards.

Observing that the plague tended to appear first on ships from the east and then spread when those ships arrived in port, trading cities began comparing notes and drawing up plans. Quarantine was first trialled in the Venetian port of Ragusa (now Dubrovnik) in 1377 – the name of the practice refers to the 40 days that suspected vessels were kept offshore to see if sailors and passengers fell sick. Within a few decades, the fundamentals of plague control had been worked out by trial and error: alongside quarantine, what we would now call notification of cases of infection, isolation of the sick, preventative sequestration by cordons sanitaires and travel restrictions, and disinfection (usually through burning the property of those infected). The main item missing from the list was carrier control. The reservoir of infection in rat fleas was not known, and systematic suppression of rat infestations was never contemplated, and presumably would have been considered impractical if it had been. Instead, people assumed that plague spread by human-to-human contagion and that rats were victims just like people.

The tools of plague containment were part of the scaffolding of the earliest administrative apparatus of the modern European state, and notably so in northern Italy. Policing the plague meant policing the people. Chroniclers of the plague wrote about the reckless indifference of poor people to the dangers of contagion, and their subversion of whatever sanitary measures were imposed upon them.[22] Daniel Defoe, in *A Journal of the Plague Year*, wrote about London:

[I]t was impossible to beat anything into the heads of the poor. They went on with the usual impetuosity of their tempers, full of outcries and lamentations when taken, but madly careless of themselves, foolhardy and obstinate, while they were well. Where they could get employment they pushed into any kind of business, the most dangerous and the most liable to infection; and if they were spoken to, their answer would be, 'I must trust to God for that; if I am taken, then I am provided for, and there is an end of me,' and the like. Or thus, 'Why, what must I do? I can't starve. I had as good have the plague as perish for want. I have no work; what could I do? I must do this or beg.'[23]

Defoe, like other literates, attributed this behaviour to ignorance, obstinacy, and fatalism. More plausibly, it was that people who lived hand-to-mouth preferred the lottery of infection to the certainty of starvation. Plague-control measures cut like scissors: one blade severed the supply of food to markets and the other cut the income from gainful employment. The price of food in the market went up just as poor people's money to buy it went down. The cause of the disease was inscrutable but the reasons for hunger were obvious to all. The science of plague control was somewhere between wrong and inexact, the motives mixed, the implementation often haphazard. Little wonder that critics condemned these measures as expensive, ineffective, and dangerous. Riots followed unemployment, high food prices, and the intrusions of gendarmes. And the plague often got through anyway.

In December 1830, the Berlin Immediate Commission presented their conclusions and plan to King Frederick Wilhelm: they backed the contagionist view, with some carefully measured reservations about how little was known about the actual causes of the disease. The king took steps to implement his operation, which was, like the Russian one, to be carried out by the army.[24]

Complicating the situation further was a more familiar threat facing the monarchs in St Petersburg, Berlin, and Vienna: rebellion in Poland. In November 1830, Polish nationalists staged an armed uprising against Russia, which had occupied the city when Poland was partitioned between Russia, Prussia, and Austria in the 1790s. The Polish rebels' target was Russia and they sensibly didn't want to fight the other occupiers at the same time, but their revolt coincided with a revolutionary uprising in France. All three kingdoms had recent memories of the Napoleonic armies that had marched across their lands. King Frederick Wilhelm mobilized his army: half his forces to his western borders in case of an attack from France, and the other half under Field Marshal August von Gneisenau to the east.

Chief of staff to Gneisenau was Clausewitz. He set aside his writing, sealed his sheaves of papers in a box, and left the military college for Berlin and then the forward headquarters of the 'Observation Army' in Posen (now Poznań). Gneisenau commanded four corps, comprising 145,000 men, which established a cordon sanitaire along Prussia's eastern border, a crescent running from Königsberg (now Kaliningrad) in the north, through Posen to Silesia – the Polish lands that had been swallowed up in the partition of Poland. They controlled that arc of land with the two objectives of preventing local Polish troops from joining the rebellion in Warsaw and enforcing the cholera exclusion zone. Clausewitz commanded forces in Danzig (now Gdańsk), the port used by Russia to resupply its troops. The royal proclamation authorized soldiers to shoot on sight anyone illegally crossing the border or violating the cordon, with penalties of imprisonment for up to 10 years for other offences.

Merchants complained loudly about loss of trade and promoted alternative medical views. Food prices jumped in Königsberg and citizens protested.[25] Gneisenau, Clausewitz, and other senior officers all had their personal views on the rationale and efficacy of the cordon. Gneisenau wrote privately that the barriers to movement and trade were 'an evil, perhaps greater than the disease itself'.[26] Clausewitz's views were more favourable. He wrote that the cordons 'reduce the evil, or rather its spread, so as [cholera] moves west, if there are always new [military] lines resisting it, it will spread into ever-thinner points and at last disappear altogether'.[27]

Cholera was not halted. The contagion marched westwards with the Russian army and reached Warsaw. It infected Polish soldiers after their early victories when they overran Russian camps and seized supplies. It sailed on Russian supply ships that docked in Danzig. And when the Poles faced defeat, they chose to surrender to the Prussians rather than the Russians and brought cholera with them too. Gneisenau himself contracted the disease and died in August, after which Clausewitz became acting commander of the Observation Army. Despite his personal views, he followed orders to wind down the operation to return to Berlin. It wasn't a victorious homecoming.

Clausewitz's brigades didn't succeed in keeping cholera out of Prussia, and the restrictions they imposed on movement and trade fomented social unrest. The historian Richard Ross concludes, '[T]he strict interventionist sanitary policies promoted by the Immediate Commission were ineffective, costly and socially destabilizing.'[28] After the campaign ended, cholera continued to infect and kill. Clausewitz left Berlin to return home to Breslau, planning to resume writing. In his study on 16 November 1831, however, he began feeling unwell, became seriously sick after midnight, and died at 9.00 a.m. the following day.

Post-Mortem on Clausewitz

Cholera was a horrible way to die, and Clausewitz's widow, Marie, provided sparse details of his last moments: 'Only around one o'clock in the morning certain symptoms of cholera revealed themselves, muscular cramps, vomiting and so on.'[29] He had a brief respite around 4.00 a.m. before the symptoms returned, worse this time, and he died shortly after daybreak. Marie wrote to a friend, 'It is a great comfort for me that at least his last moments were peaceful and painless but there was still something heart-breaking in the manner, in the tone with which he exhaled his last breath; because it was as if he had shuddered life away as a heavy burden.'[30] She was calmed by the doctor's opinion that his death could be attributed more to 'the state of his nerves' than the disease.

Marie's husband didn't meet with death in the manner he would have hoped. Clausewitz had been one of the leaders in building a new Prussian army, which was an exercise in myth-making as much as in professional training and organization. The old army – crushed by Napoleon at the battle of Jena-Auerstedt in 1806 – had been commanded by aristocrats who inherited military ranks along with their feudal titles, and about half of its soldiers had been mercenaries. In the new army, military service was a duty to the nation. The king and his generals, along with songwriters, artists, and churchmen, nourished the 'cult of the fallen soldier'. Death in battle was depicted in royal statements, poems, songs, and paintings as a heroic sacrifice for the fatherland, and every man who 'fell on the field of honour' was commemorated in a plaque in his local church.[31] The newly minted Iron Cross was awarded to those displaying great courage, including posthumously to those heroes who didn't return. Dying from a diarrhoeal disease did not fit this script. Marie's correspondents would have known the disgusting realities of cholera, but all would have joined in discreet silence over her husband's last hours.

Clausewitz's slightly older contemporary, the philosopher Georg Hegel, profoundly influenced how Europeans thought about death. His interpretation of Sophocles' *Antigone* not only redefined the genre of tragedy but also helped establish the 19th-century vision of a 'beautiful death', especially in its feminine form.[32] In the classic, high-philosophy version, the tragic hero embraces death by taking control of the manner of dying, transforming it into a meaningful culmination of life. Hegel, too, died of cholera, just three days before Clausewitz. Out of respect for his social standing, the Berlin city authorities waived the requirement that he be buried at night in a special cholera cemetery.[33]

In the popular version, the 'beautiful death' also became a Romantic feminine aesthetic, realized through the pallid and drawn figures of women's bodies.[34] Sickening of consumption (tuberculosis) was an artful way of life and even a fashionable death. Tragic suicide was another. Cholera, with its total loss of control of bodily functions culminating in continuing twitching in the minutes after death, was the irreconcilable antithesis of this. For Marie von Clausewitz and her social circle, the dread of cholera was sharpened by the horrible manner of one's dying.

On War was the most exhaustive and coherent exploration of the theory and practice of warfare to date. Marie's contribution, which went beyond compiling and copy-editing the published version to include some of the theoretical formulations, has only recently been recognized.[35] Clausewitz's theory of war revolves around two definitions: war is 'an act of violence intended to compel our opponent to fulfil our will' and 'the mere continuation of politics by other means'.[36] *On War* analyses the logic of escalation towards 'absolute war': 'War is an act of violence pushed to its utmost bounds; as one side dictates the law to the other, there arises a sort of reciprocal action, which logically must lead to an extreme.'[37] Scholars have debated whether Clausewitz was simply describing this logic or celebrating it. The German historian Hans Rothfels decried it as reducing strategy to a 'rage of numbers'.[38]

Clausewitz's writings on war are considered comprehensive, but it is striking how little he has to say about disease. He writes about the 'infinity of petty circumstances' such as problems of broken roads, lame horses, and bad weather, all as elements of the 'friction' of war. He writes that 'War is the province of uncertainty: three-fourths of those things upon which action in War must be calculated, are hidden more or less in the clouds of great uncertainty.'[39] Disease is implicit in the 'fog of war', but the only explicit mention comes in his chapter on how to sustain an assembled army over a period of time:

> Fatigue, exertion, and privation constitute in War a special principle of destruction, not essentially belonging to

contest, but more or less inseparably bound up with it . . .
[In strategy] their influence is not only always very considerable, but often quite decisive. It is not at all uncommon for a
victorious Army to lose many more by sickness than on the
field of battle.[40]

That's it: a tremendous caveat mentioned casually in passing.
It is as though disease was simply a reality of life and death
that should be fatalistically accepted and about which little
or nothing could be done. Perhaps Clausewitz would have
expanded on this short passage after returning from his mission in Posen; undoubtedly, he would have welcomed more
systematic military medicine. Would he also have added a
chapter on 'war on disease' to *On War*? This is not likely.
At that time, Europe's royalty often used troops to suppress
civil disturbances, and Clausewitz doesn't consider these
either. In the same way, the Observation Army's operation
on the Polish border wasn't a 'war' but rather the kind of
distasteful but unavoidable use of troops to maintain civil
order. For sure, Clausewitz would have made a first-rate
public health planner and administrator and might have used
the occasional warlike metaphor such as an 'attack' by the
disease. But we can be confident that he wouldn't have considered it proper war.

Cholera's New Order

Cholera caused disruption and dismay: political, geographical, and scientific. After Berlin and Danzig, the pandemic
rolled across Europe, apparently unstoppable. It faded and
then reappeared in the 1840s, more ship-borne this time.
Physicians, princes, merchants, city planners, and revolutionaries debated what had caused this calamity and why
Europe was so powerless to stop it. No one could agree,
even in Paris, where the investigations were more thorough and detailed than anywhere else. The new plague was

simply too capricious. It wasn't just Europeans who were baffled: Hindu belief and ritual had long incorporated diseases such as smallpox into its cosmos, but not cholera.[41] Neither authority nor tradition had a prescription, so necessity issued a charter for experimentation and debate. Because the answers – and even the terms of the debate and the methods for reaching answers – weren't agreed, the verdict could change from one year to the next, and back again. The exchanges were often polemical; as is common in the wake of a defeat, the politics were rancorous, bad-tempered, and decided by something other than a rational and dispassionate assessment of the evidence.[42] Unencumbered by the reductionism of germ theory, unconstrained by professional or academic boundaries which were yet to be erected, observers put forward all manner of theories for epidemics and for epidemic diseases. Later on, an 'epidemic' came to mean an aggregation of cases of a particular disease, a simple positivist framework that filtered out the social element. Over the course of the century, as positivistic microbiology gained power and reputation, it became unfashionable to think of an epidemic as a social event.

By the 1860s, when the fourth pandemic followed the same paths, European city planners, sanitation and hygiene advocates, merchants, and port authorities had hit on a workable system of protecting themselves against cholera. They didn't 'follow the science', because the science, such as it was, led in different directions. Some of the 'right' measures were adopted for the 'wrong' reasons. And in fact, consensus on contagionism, reinvented as a microscopic germ theory, came only in the 1880s, when Europe's practical problem of cholera had already been solved.

In the meantime, there was a drumbeat of fear. It was fear of sudden and ignominious death followed by hasty midnight burial in a mass grave. It was fear of the mayhem of the mob, of revolutionary uprisings spreading like a forest fire. It was fear of the fragility of civilization. Every literate European was familiar with Edward Gibbon's *The Decline and Fall of the*

Roman Empire and his account of the pestilence and famine that ravaged the reign of the Emperor Justinian.[43] Many would have visited Rome, which in classical times, as its ruins showed, was as large as any city in contemporary Europe and considerably more sophisticated. Early 19th-century Europe was on the cusp of the great acceleration – the take-off into sustained growth – but that wasn't clear to those at the time. Equally possible was a historical cycle in which the future was a return to barbarism. The drumbeat was also fear of the unknown. The grammar of cholera was incomprehensible. Counter-plague measures hadn't worked, which had discredited the contagionist theory, and 'anti-contagionism' had the intellectual edge. In the depths of dismay and disarray in the 1830s, the more credible and socially progressive scientists criticized contagionist practices as simplistic and unscientific.[44] And they did so in a properly rational and targeted way: they were *cholera* anti-contagionists and didn't dismiss contagion *per se*. Some miasmatists believed that there was an infectious element in the air, and all recognized that diseases such as syphilis, smallpox, and measles were transmissible in some manner.

The empirical problem with early 19th-century contagionism was that it simply couldn't explain why outbreaks began and ended when and where they did. At that time, contagionism was based on the idea of the direct transmission of an inanimate poison by touch. For plague, typhus, yellow fever, and the new Asiatic cholera, this couldn't explain the vagaries of transmission.[45] Each of these diseases seemed sometimes to jump from place to place without a discernible human chain of contagion while nurses and carers were often oddly unaffected by them. But anti-contagionists also couldn't agree on what caused cholera or what could stop it. Did it originate as a miasma in India and then spread through human agency, taking hold in local soils? Could it be blown by the wind? Why were low-lying places more susceptible than higher altitudes? Why did outbreaks start in ports? What they agreed upon was that it was complicated.

The anti-contagionists' philosophical point was that ideas of contagion had been around for millennia, had been adapted from the Bible to medical practice, and had never been subjected to scientific scrutiny. To understand this from the viewpoint of the 21st century, we must suspend our belief in germ theory and see dirt in the pre-modern sense, not as a potential carrier of pathogens, but as things in the wrong place. Concepts of contagion, contamination, and uncleanliness originated in worldviews that long preceded scientific understanding of disease. Two hundred years ago, Christian preachers would present the prohibitions in the Book of Leviticus *in toto*, including the ban on eating shellfish, on men having contact with menstruating women, and on cross-breeding animals or mixing the seeds of different plants in the same field. They wouldn't sort them into some individual ancient rules that made hygienic sense and others that didn't. They were closer to the original pre-modern understanding of those biblical rules as a comprehensive worldview, in which concepts of pollution and transgression, wholeness and purity, provided the mental scaffolding for natural, social, and spiritual categories.[46]

Today, we like to think that medical practice is based upon scientific evidence, including the results of biological experiments and data compiled from controlled trials. Before the 19th century, there were indeed pioneering physicians and statisticians of health who thought this way, but they were a small and informal cosmopolitan club of individuals. The established medical profession was more like a masonic lodge whose members practised a mixture of craft and performance on the authority of tradition.[47] Over the 2,300 years since Hippocrates, European doctors applied remedies that were more likely to kill than to heal. Bloodletting was so common that the instrument used for opening veins, the lancet, symbolized the profession (and the oldest and most prestigious medical journal is named after it even today). Surgeons rarely sterilized surgical equipment and often didn't even wash their hands properly, so that it was much safer for a woman to deliver her baby at home attended by a midwife than to go to hospital, where she ran a serious risk of cross-infection from her surgeon's hands or forceps. The history of medical progress includes tragic cases of pioneers who were ridiculed for their discoveries, including promoting basic hygiene. It wasn't until the 1860s that the scientific revolution at long last reformed medical practice.

One new practice stood out as an exception: inoculation against smallpox. This practice was introduced to Europeans from China via the Ottoman Empire, and to Americans via Africa. In both cases, it was people outside the medical establishment who were responsible: the wife of the British ambassador to the court of the Ottoman Sultan in Constantinople, Lady Mary Wortley Montagu, and an African slave in Massachusetts known to history only by the name Onesimus, given to him by his American master (who is remembered, but not in this book). The first procedure adopted was 'variolation': the injection of infected material from the scabs of a person suffering mild smallpox into a healthy person with the aim of inducing a mild form of the disease. Asians and Africans had learned that this bestowed lifelong immunity.

Variolation was perilous. In some people, it induced a severe case of smallpox and between 1 and 2 per cent of them died. The comparable figure was 30 per cent when the disease was contracted naturally. This is where mathematicians enter the story, refining the concept and measurement of risk. There were two different debates on risk. The French statistician Daniel Bernouilli calculated that the comprehensive inoculation of a population would increase life expectancy by two years.[48] A rival statistician, Jean Le Rond d'Alembert, posed the question of risk from the viewpoint of individual choice rather than aggregate population welfare: under what circumstances could a person make the decision in a fair and rational way, for themselves or their family?[49] D'Alembert doubted whether a matter of public policy should be determined on the basis of probabilities.

The second debate arose because the procedure could cause not only individual sickness but outbreaks too. John Haygarth, an English country doctor who in 1793 proposed a nationwide campaign of inoculation to eradicate smallpox from the British Isles, developed a set of rules that would minimize this danger. For example, he said patients should be quarantined after variolation. Haygarth wasn't liked by his peers. Physicians rejected his ideas that medical practice might cause accidental epidemics and that physicians should be regulated by calculations of systematic public health.[50] Soon after, when Edward Jenner discovered that inoculation with cowpox – vaccination – could achieve immunity in almost total safety, Haygarth and his rules were forgotten.

Nonetheless, applying statistical method to disease control promised a revolution in public health. After cholera ravaged Paris in 1832, men of science and mathematics conducted the most thorough investigation of the age into the correlates of infection. The only indisputable finding was that it targeted the poor. Otherwise, the immense compendium of statistical material served as an arsenal for contending theoreticians to pursue their academic combat.[51] In the 1830s and 1840s, the different medical-scientific camps aligned broadly with political programmes: authoritarian centralists tended to be contagionists while liberal free traders and free thinkers were anti-contagionists.[52] Doctors could be at home in either camp, as their practices were curative and could accommodate either theory, and those with high social standing followed whatever the establishment decreed. Physicians who wanted their profession to be independent and self-regulating mostly sided with the forward-thinking anti-contagionists.

Thirty years later, contagionists and anti-contagionists had each sharpened their arguments. Louis Pasteur (1822–95), the father of modern germ theory, introduced scientific methods to medicine in a revolutionary manner. He debated with his fellow scientists in Paris – sometimes in a collegial manner, sometimes not – over which was more important, the microbe or the milieu. In Germany, the protagonists were Robert Koch (1843–1910) and Max von Pettenkofer (1818–1901), whose rivalry began and ended over cholera, so they will be reintroduced as exemplars of the different camps later on. Strikingly absent from these debates was the theory of evolution by natural selection. Charles Darwin published *On the Origin of Species* in 1859, which provoked vigorous public debate, but its insights were not applied to the study of pathogens for a hundred years.

The Streets of London

History was made in the streets of Europe's fast-expanding cities. Humble but angry people marched and rioted, petitioned and set up barricades, and occasionally seized control of alleyways, boulevards, and squares. It is notable that the second, third, and fourth pandemics each ran through Europe at moments of revolution and war: the 1830 Parisian barricades and Polish rebellion; the 1848 'springtime of the peoples'; and the wars and upheavals of the 1860s that culminated in the Paris Commune. But turn the lens to bring into focus the details of each upheaval and cholera's correlates become blurry: there is also hunger, unemployment, and the plotting of revolutionaries to take into account.[53] A lot of other things were going on, and the reason why many histories of the era don't mention cholera at all isn't ignorance or denial, but because these were decades of social change, economic upheaval, and political ferment without precedent. Cholera was one element in the intellectual and political disorder of the time. It seemed to ignite lawlessness wherever it struck. The St Petersburg riots scared the authorities, not only in Russia, and were a big reason why the anti-contagionists got a sympathetic hearing. French reactionaries saw the threat: infection was subversion, and policing the disease was about policing the people. François Delaporte quotes one, questioning whether Paris suffered the disease because of natural transmission: 'No, [it spread] rather by revolutionary infection, which progresses in the same way, which erupts without good reason. . . . Cholera, like revolution, must be eradicated at the source.'[54] Contemporaries started talking about 'cholera riots'.[55] Meanwhile, ordinary people also drew their own conclusions, and most often it was that they shouldn't trust the authorities. Among their accusations were that physicians were deliberately poisoning people, that hospitals were places where doctors experimented on the bodies of the dead, that rulers were using the disease to clear the poor neighbourhoods of cities, and that the epidemic was induced to solve the problem of unemployment by eliminating surplus labour.

Cholera epidemics hit hardest in the new industrial cities, where jerry-built housing had been built apace without even rudimentary sanitation, and the older commercial centres, where medieval quarters were grossly overcrowded. It was a disease of capitalist industry and commerce. When it struck, the wealthy fled the city to their country homes, leaving the poor to suffer. We might expect the self-appointed vanguard of the emergent proletariat to have identified the people's health as a front in their newly declared class war, and marshal their intellectual and propaganda weapons accordingly. Friedrich Engels, in his 1845 book *The Condition of the Working Class in England*, documented the discrepancies in nutrition, health, life expectancy, and height between the working poor and the bourgeoisie, attributing the deprivations of the former to the greed of the latter. He reprised the popular opinion that the accidents, illnesses, and privations that shortened the lives of the poor were 'social murder'. But Engels missed cholera entirely. He added this bare paragraph to the 1892 reprint:

> Again, the repeated visitations of cholera, typhus, small-pox, and other epidemics have shown the British bourgeois the urgent necessity of sanitation in his towns and cities, if he wishes to save himself and family from falling victims to

such diseases. Accordingly, the most crying abuses described in this book have either disappeared or have been made less conspicuous.[56]

Engels, it seems, quietly conceded that epidemic control was a bourgeois science, and an effective one to boot. For the communists, war and class war were the locomotives of history, and contagious microbes were merely passengers. As the historian Samuel Cohn observes, this is a baffling surrender of a political battlefield where Marxists could have outflanked their class enemies. 'An analysis of cholera and its social consequences did not enter any of Marx's works published in his lifetime,' he notes, 'and he appears to have been oblivious to any manifestations of its social protest and class struggle ... despite these events sparking crowds estimated as high as 30,000, taking control of cities (even if only briefly), murdering governors, mayors, judges, physicians, pharmacists, and nurses, destroying factories and towns.'[57] The explanation is that 19th-century communists were firm believers in the material sciences and technological progress. They didn't value folk wisdom or traditional ways of life; Marx dismissed the peasantry as a 'sack of potatoes' and the lowest stratum of urban workers as the 'rabble' or lumpenproletariat. The communists wouldn't challenge sanitary engineering or microscopy any more than they would denigrate the steam engine.

Other radicals saw the connection between politics and disease more clearly and were determined to act. The leading exemplar is Rudolph Virchow (1821–1902), a remarkable German physician and politician who was one of the first doctors to become an activist political reformer. As well as a pioneer of cellular biology, Virchow was an anthropologist (an early critic of the racist leanings of physical anthropology), and his painstaking inquiry into an epidemic of 'hunger typhus' in Silesia – one of the provinces where Clausewitz's Observation Army had deployed a few years earlier – led him to argue passionately that the causes lay in poverty, lack of education, and the absence of democracy.[58] He made the case that medical interventions on their own had little value, but rather social advancement through education, democracy, and prosperity was needed to end epidemic disease. Virchow joined the 1848 uprisings with the slogan, 'Medicine is a social science, and politics is nothing but medicine at scale.'[59] As leader of the Progressive Party in parliament, Virchow fervently opposed militarism and voted against Chancellor Otto von Bismarck's 1865 bill for increasing spending on the army.[60]

While Virchow was campaigning for social reform as the cure for epidemic disease in Berlin, Karl Marx was lodging at 28 Dean Street, London, each day walking to the rotunda of the Reading Room at the British Museum, 11 minutes in each direction (according to Google Maps, and the streets haven't changed). Had he chosen to walk five minutes in the opposite direction, he would have arrived at a water pump on Broad Street, which was the epicentre of a cholera outbreak that killed more than five hundred people over three weeks in August–September 1854. It was a localized but fierce outbreak that spread terror in the neighbourhood, and also prompted a seminal and fascinating investigation into the cause of the disease. The cholera didn't quite reach Dean Street – the closest affected house (on Meard Street) was a block away. In a letter to Engels, Marx wrote somewhat coarsely: '[A]s Soho is a choice district for cholera, the mob is croaking right and left (e.g. an average of 3 per house in Broad Street).'[61]

Had Marx continued on his hypothetical walk to Broad Street, he would have passed the church of St Luke's. (It no longer exists.) Its curate was the Reverend Henry Whitehead (1825–96), a man with more respect for the poor families amongst whom he lived. Whitehead's walks precisely circumscribed the outbreak:

If a person were to start from the western end of Broad Street, and, after traversing its whole length on the south

side from west to east, to return as far as the brewery, and
then, going down Hopkins Street, along Husband Street,
and up New Street, to end by walking through Pulteney
Court, he would pass successively forty-five houses, of
which only six escaped without a death during the recent
outburst of cholera in that neighbourhood. According to
a calculation based upon the last census, those forty-five
houses contained a population of about 1,000. Out of that
number 104 perished by the pestilence.[62]

The curate became an assiduous practitioner of the humble
craft of people's epidemiology. His pedestrian language and
method – the pamphlet from which I have just quoted runs to
17 pages of similar details – could not be in greater contrast
with the ambitious dialectics of his intellectual neighbour.
Whitehead knew his parishioners one by one and had gained
their confidence in such a way that he could ask them simple
but intimate questions about their everyday lives, in particular, from where they obtained their drinking water, and how
they disposed of their excrement.[63]

Whitehead was the Dr Watson to the Sherlock Holmes
of cholera's most famous disease detective, John Snow. For
some years, Snow had been convinced that, first of all, the
miasma theory of cholera didn't hold water (as it were). Snow
was London's leading anaesthetist and an expert on gases and
how they affected human beings. In his view, the carefully
compiled meteorological tables that were used in evidence
for the airborne theory of cholera transmission were a pile
of useless data (the obvious diarrhoeal disease-related metaphors aren't printable). Secondly, Snow had noticed how
cholera cases tracked the pumped water supplies of different companies and had been working on a careful statistical
comparison of this for several years. As a vegetarian, he had
started drinking only filtered water because of the living
organisms visible to the eye in London's water.[64] When the
Soho outbreak erupted, he suspended all his other inquir-
ies as well as his medical practice to investigate. He asked

the curate to join him. Whitehead was at first sceptical of Snow's theory, but was converted as the two went, patient-by-patient and house-by-house. Shoe-leather epidemiology is applied social work or social anthropology. Some people who fell sick did so because they sent their children to get water from the Broad Street pump, whereas a group of older widows who didn't have children to run errands drank water delivered from another pump, and escaped.[65] The workers at the nearby brewery proudly refused to drink water at all and not one of them succumbed. Snow's detective work demonstrated that cholera was transmitted by contaminated water, and by those who attended to the sick failing to follow hygienic practices. His natural experiment, using the streets of London as his laboratory, are seminal to epidemiology as a science.

Snow is rightly celebrated as a hero of the discipline and of epidemic prevention. The story of how he diligently tracked down the still-invisible culprit for the Soho outbreak is the template for all subsequent disease detective stories. Variants of this detective story are written for every epidemic, whether cases of salmonella from a village hall buffet or the outbreak of a novel coronavirus in East Asia. Broad Street is where it all began. At the time, however, neither Snow nor his detractors made use of metaphors of police and criminal culprits, or soldiers defending against invisible enemies – at least not in any systematic way. In a rare use of warlike imagery, Whitehead compared the cholera outbreak to a mine exploding under a city's ramparts, 'revealing to the startled population of an ill-managed city the peril of [their] position'.[66] Until a recent book by Steven Johnson, Whitehead's role was almost entirely overlooked in the annals of health science. This prefigures a recurrent blind-spot in public health: the public is conceived as the aggregation upon which disease and policy work, not as agents of change.

Snow died in 1858, before he was vindicated. He and Whitehead toiled alone, scorned by the London authorities and the public health experts of the day. The editors of *The Lancet* excoriated Snow as a charlatan and didn't mention his cholera work in his obituary (the journal reversed its position in 1866). The government adopted a version of miasmatism that blamed cholera (along with sundry other diseases) on noxious vapours. London was a smelly city and becoming smellier as its population grew faster than its sanitation. Excrement piled up in cesspits, cellars, and the streets; travellers from out of town could smell the city before they could see it. The sanitation movement, headed by Edwin Chadwick, pressed for employers and municipalities to take responsibility for the conditions of their workers and residents, and campaigned for clean air, piped water, and sewage disposal. Chadwick's greatest policy achievement was the 1848 Public Health Act; his greatest monument was the London sewers designed by Joseph Bazalgette, which would rank as one of the wonders of the industrial era were they visible above ground for the public to admire. The Thames Embankment was built to cover the sewers underneath. The investments in public sanitation inspired by Chadwick and built by Bazalgette brought many benefits, but ironically, in its first years, the world's most ambitious plumbing scheme pumped sewers into the river Thames, which had the immediate effect of spreading waterborne pathogens. Cholera bacilli that would previously have been confined to a neighbourhood cesspit were now delivered straight to the city's water supply. This problem disappeared when the entire scheme was completed in the 1860s. Huge sewage filtration plants were constructed and the river was cleaned up. London's cholera problem was first worsened and then solved by the massive application of technology according to a theory that was wrong.

Speaking to a parliamentary inquiry following what was to be London's last cholera outbreak in 1866, the statistician William Farr – a late convert to Snow's waterborne thesis – pointed out that water's innocence had long been maintained by water companies, but air retained no defence counsel to plead on its behalf.[67] The communists missed that story, just as they missed the way in which disease was a selective affliction of empire.

Cholera's Empire

A contemporary apologist for the British Empire, the historian Niall Ferguson, has celebrated what he describes as the six 'killer apps' whereby European civilization triumphed: competition, science, property, medicine, consumption, and hard work.[68] Subjects of empire might have compiled a different and more literal list of 'killer apps'. Let's start with cholera. Colonialism – arguably the original culprit for pandemic cholera – was modestly redesigned to manage the disease, and not transformed so as to eliminate it.

In the 1860s, Britain managed to square the circle of its mercantile interest in free trade and the brute fact that some form of contagionism was clearly correct. The government did this in a similar way to London's overflowing waste: it applied enough resources to the problem to ensure that it would go away, regardless of which scientific theory was correct. From the start, the contagionism controversy had never been just about the science, it was also about quarantine, which meant that it was about free and uninterrupted maritime trade. In 1831, a correspondent in *The Lancet* opined that the contagion theory was 'a humbug got up for the restriction of our commerce'.[69] With the anti-contagionist tide of that decade, Europe dismantled its quarantines and cordons sanitaires. Even Marseilles, which had the most vigilant quarantine and isolation statutes on its books after the 1720 plague outbreak, relaxed them in 1835. Some controls were then reintroduced, especially after the first international sanitary conference in Paris in 1851. At the third conference, in Constantinople in 1866, convened shortly after the fourth pandemic reached Europe, delegates endorsed contagionist theories.

Just as significant was the Suez Canal. When construction began in 1859, it promised that the single most important artery for Britain's colonial trade would pass through a French-administered canal to the Mediterranean instead of around the Cape of Good Hope. The shipping time from London to Bombay would be cut in half. As the digging progressed, British importers feared that the canal authorities, backed by the Constantinople cholera commission, would insist that ships could be kept at sea for the then-standard 20 to 65 days' quarantine on suspicion of cholera. London's solution was to develop what became known as the 'English system' of medical inspection and surveillance as an alternative to quarantine. It was run by Britain's Port Sanitary Authorities. A medical inspector boarded every incoming ship to certify whether there were visible signs of cholera or other listed diseases on board. If so, the ship was disinfected, and anyone on board with suspicious symptoms was transferred to an isolation hospital. Any other crew and passengers who displayed no symptoms were monitored after landing by domestic health officers.[70] It accorded with the laissez-faire agenda of the shipping merchants. But while old-style quarantine was simple to enforce, this new system needed an expensive and complicated bureaucracy both at the seaport and domestically.[71] Britain was rich enough to do this, but not many other states could muster the means.

The administration of India was a different matter. In 1857, there was a huge rebellion against foreign rule and its exactions. The so-called 'mutiny' was suppressed with mass killing, and in the aftermath the British government abolished the East India Company and set up an imperial government directly responsible to Whitehall. The purpose of controlling India didn't change, though: it was to profit the metropolis, through cheap cotton exports to Lancashire and direct subsidy to the Treasury. Meanwhile, India was to pay for its own imperial government. The British Raj wasn't ready to spend the amount of money necessary to replicate the 'English system' in India, especially the component of urban sanitation. Colonial medical officers were well aware that plans for the territory would worsen the problem of cholera, not alleviate it. Notably, irrigated farming schemes were expanded to grow cotton for export. These were constructed cheaply. One design shortcut was economizing on drainage channels, without which water stagnated in pools and swamps, providing new habitats for the *Vibrio cholerae*.[72] Railways were recognized as a means of transmission: we know this because army medical officers provided detailed recommendations for how to contain an outbreak on a train and make sure that sick soldiers' excreta weren't dumped on the tracks.[73] But this topic never got attention in British India. Rather, Indians were accused of being unhygienic and resistant to education.

If we are adding up numbers, the single biggest imperial killer was famine. From the beginnings of the East India Company's forays into Bengal, famine was its constant companion, with starvation intensifying in step with company profits. Little changed with direct imperial rule. Officials were enamoured of the thesis attributed to the Reverend Thomas Malthus, a kind of demographic fury. Malthus's 'principle of population' was that the number of people would increase geometrically (2, 4, 8, 16, etc.), whereas food production was destined to expand only arithmetically (2, 3, 4, 5, etc.) until such point that 'gigantic inevitable Famine' would strike down population to a level in line with food supply. Malthus himself toyed with this formulation only briefly, in the first (1798) edition of his *Essay on Population*, and although he was later appointed to be professor of political economy at the East India Company's college at Haileybury, he never imposed this doctrine on his students. Nonetheless, British officials in India embraced it and insisted that population growth was a greater evil than famine. Parsimonious spending on famine relief was a more esteemed virtue than saving lives that would, presumably, be lost anyway at some future point.[74] Cholera enters the picture because the famine relief policy of providing assistance only to those who had the right combination of destitute circumstances and willingness to labour on public works (often digging irrigation ditches) meant that hungry people congregated in huge relief shelters, which had little or no organized sanitation. It is no surprise that cholera accompanied food crisis time and again.[75]

It wasn't ignorance that led London to design different cholera-control policies in Britain and India. What happened was that the Colonial Office decided to wash its hands of science-based public health. In a little-observed about-face, brought to light by the historian Sheldon Watts, the imperial government in India took an explicitly denialist position on the science of epidemic disease. In 1867, a sanitary commissioner named James M. Cuningham completed a routine report into a recent cholera outbreak that analysed the problem and recommended responses in line with the consensus view that the disease was caused by a 'poison' carried by human beings. Before it was published, however, he was instructed by his superiors to suppress it and reverse his position.[76] Cuningham complied and as a reward he was promoted. Thereafter, reports on epidemic diseases in India were published only in summary form and research was stymied. A few years later, when another sanitary officer proposed reforms that included bringing clean water to villages and providing classes in hygiene, Cuningham drafted the official reply, paraphrased thus:

It was beyond government's resources to increase the comforts of so large a proportion of its population. ... [I]t is certain that the attempt to do so would lead to a very large increase in the number [of people] to be dealt with [and that] so long as poverty existed, its concomitants must be accepted as inevitable however painful they may be to contemplate.[77]

Between 1817 and 1865, cholera killed about 15 million Indians. Between 1865 and 1947, it killed 23 million.[78] Its grim reaper didn't slacken his rhythm. For 30 years after the last cholera deaths in Britain, perfidious Albion maintained an entirely different set of doctrines for cholera control – as well as for respect for basic humanity – east of Suez. The Indian policy couldn't be sustained intellectually, so details were suppressed and practices were justified through a kind of epidemiological orientalism, claiming that disease worked differently for Asians.

Meanwhile, London adopted an amalgam of measures to stop cholera travelling. It helped that Britain took control of the Suez Canal. The Egyptian viceroy borrowed from London banks to pay for the digging of the canal. A few years after it was opened in 1869, he began running into arrears. Her Majesty's Government called time on the debt and repossessed the defaulter's real estate by force of arms – an invasion. France protested but could do little, and its prized canal was now in British hands along with the enforcement of any agreed quarantine regulations, or lack thereof. The French public had contributed money to build a towering bronze statue of an Egyptian lady, designed by Frédéric Auguste Bartholdi, holding a flaming torch. 'Egypt bringing light to Asia' was to stand at the entrance to the Suez Canal. She would have presided over a quarantine station for ships headed in the opposite, westerly-bound voyage. Bartholdi's monumental sculpture was renamed the 'Statue of Liberty' and shipped to New York instead, where it stood welcoming those immigrants who had passed their quarantine screening at Swinburne and Hoffman Islands in the outer harbour.

Another way the 'English system' worked was that France's more assertive imperial health policies suited Britain's trade. The immediate alarm was an outbreak of cholera affecting pilgrims on the Hajj to Mecca in 1865. That year, one in six of the 90,000 pilgrims died. Fear of cholera reaching Europe by way of the Red Sea 'succeeded in uniting rival European powers in a concerted politique sanitaire whose objective was regulation of the life of Western Arabia and, no less, the most sacred ritual of Islam, the Hajj'.[79] France took the lead, depicting cholera as an 'invasion' from Asia, which justified pushing the outer ramparts of Europe's sanitary frontier further into Ottoman-ruled lands. Western European health officers were stationed in Cairo and Constantinople with the authority to control the westward departure of ships. Ostensibly sovereign, the Ottoman Empire was losing authority over its ports on the pretext of disease control. The historian Patrick Zylberman has described this as 'preemptive intervention' in the eastern Mediterranean and beyond.[80] The Ottoman state was the 'sick man of Europe' in two senses of the phrase, and the imperialist predators were already sinking their teeth into its weakening body.

France's own *mission civilisatrice* had scientific medicine at its ideological centre.[81] Hubert Lyautey, the French general who conquered Morocco, portrayed public health this way: '[T]he physician, if he understands his role, is the most effective of our agents of penetration and pacification.'[82] But its practice had similar double standards to Britain's: the medical officers of the colonial Pasteur Institutes were tasked with impressive but cheap campaigns of mass vaccination, while the infrastructure of sanitation and social medicine was built only within the hexagon of France itself. The main function of tropical medicine was keeping the white man healthy so he could seize colonial territories, for profit and prestige. Along with that theft came an imperial classification: of territory, plants and animals, races and tribes, and microbes.

Declaring War on Disease

Germany was a latecomer to tropical empire. Having unified the German-speaking lands between Poland and the Rhine, and defeated France, the kaiser started to stake out his 'place in the sun'. It was a matter of status as much as land and resources and his eyes were on Africa, the last continent where the white man had not drawn his lines on the map. While the imperial staff began planning to convene Europe's ministers in Berlin, an opportunity arose to claim to another parcel of the natural world.

In 1882, it became clear that a fifth cholera pandemic was under way. Germany's leading microbiologist, Robert Koch, travelled to Egypt to apply his skills to identifying the pathogen responsible. He wasn't aware that the Florentine microbiologist Filippo Pacini had already done this in 1854 as the latter had no patron to broadcast his discovery.[83] Koch arrived in Alexandria in August 1883 and found a French team led by Émile Roux, a close associate of Louis Pasteur, already at work on the same task – they did in fact isolate the bacillus but couldn't prove whether it was cause or correlate of the disease. Koch also found it in post-mortem examinations, but had the same doubts about its role. Koch and his team then followed the bacteria's own voyage in reverse to Calcutta, where they repeated their investigations. On 7 January 1884, Koch sent a message to Berlin that he had successfully cultured the microbe, followed a few weeks later by another dispatch explaining his conviction that the bacillus was truly the causal agent and adding that it was 'a little bent, like a comma'.[84] His message wasn't addressed to his scientific colleagues but to the German Secretary of State for the Interior, an indication that his mission was political as well as medical.

The British colonial authorities weren't impressed with Koch. They claimed that they knew far more about the disease and the local conditions in which it thrived than this upstart German. Sir Joseph Fayrer, 1st Baronet FRS FRSE FRCS FRCP KCSI LLD,[85] Surgeon General of the Imperial Government of India, wrote that 'he could not believe that a small material entity [i.e. a microbe] had much to do with those vast epidemic waves which depopulated districts.'[86] Under Fayrer's guidance, two British experts sailed for Calcutta, arriving after the epidemic had passed, to evaluate Koch's claims. They discounted the germ theory in favour of 60 years' worth of accumulated wisdom from British observers, and their report concluded by repeating 'the inutility of sanitary cordons and quarantine restrictions which are also injurious by creating alarm and preventing the furtherance of valuable sanitary measures'.[87]

British colonialists much preferred the theories of the German sanitationist Max von Pettenkofer and continued to invoke them for the next decade.[88] Pettenkofer is little known today but 150 years ago he was Europe's most eminent chemist and anti-contagionist. He championed medical research, advocated clean air and urban sanitation, mentored dozens of students, and founded the Munich Institute of Hygiene – a model for similar schools in Baltimore and London, where his name is inscribed on the frieze of the London School of Hygiene and Tropical Medicine, along with 22 other white male pioneers of the field. In the folk history of medicine, all these achievements count for naught: he is instead the villain whose obstinacy led him to the fatal mistake of opposing the waterborne theory of cholera transmission.[89] But despite this, and despite the way he was cited by colonial rulers, we should look more kindly on Pettenkofer. He was trying to develop a theory of disease that combined pathogen, environment, and individual in what we would now call a complex multi-factorial interaction. His theory was that a combination of several conditions was needed for an epidemic: a specific germ referred to as disease agent (x), and local and seasonal conditions especially affecting the soil (y) to create the 'cholera miasma' (z), which would, depending on individual proclivity, cause disease.[90] Among the subclassifications of scientists at the time, he would be called a 'contingent anti-contagionist' who combined elements from miasmatism, localism, and contagionism. His postulates included:

> 7: The nature of x, y and z is so far unknown but one may assume, with a scientific probability bordering on certainty, that all three are of organic nature and that x, at least, is an organized germ or body.
>
> . . .

9: The facts support the assumption that x can feed itself and maybe considerably multiply in the human body, e.g., in the intestine, but the human body is in the case of cholera only the showplace of the effect of z, and cannot produce z alone, if x does not enter in contact with y.[91]

Pettenkofer asked many of the right questions about infectious disease outbreaks. He tirelessly advocated for clean air, clean water, and clean streets, and his views were perfectly compatible with water purification. Where he erred was in insisting that cholera wasn't contracted through water and that there was no purpose in isolating people with the disease, just as it wouldn't make sense to quarantine people poisoned by a toxic gas leak. Pettenkofer wasn't just a scientist, he was a publicist for public health, and – for a while – the most influential adviser in Germany's Cholera Commission.[92] In 1876, he took the post of chief scientific adviser to Bismarck.

Koch had a different cast of character. He was a micro-bacteriologist who zeroed in on finding microbes. Koch's proposition was just x: the singular culprit for each disease was a germ. The aetiology of infectious disease was distilled to an invisible invader that could be picked out by a trained microbiologist. Koch's first scientific achievement was identifying the lifecycle of anthrax, but because he was unable to specify the exact causal mechanism in the disease, he fell back upon the metaphor of 'host' and 'parasite'.[93] It was an inspired innovation and it is easy to forget that it began as a metaphor. In the meantime, Koch refined bacteriological method. Along with his mentor, Jakob Henle, he developed four postulates for certifying a microscopic pathogen as the cause of a disease. According to the Henle–Koch postulates, the microbiologist had first to identify the suspected microbe in all infected individuals; then it should be grown in a culture in the laboratory; third, he had to use the microbe extracted from this culture to infect an experimental animal and observe it sicken with similar symptoms; and finally the scientist had to isolate the same microbe in the sick or deceased animal. The experiment had to be repeatable. This method came to define both pathogen and disease.

Tuberculosis fitted. When Koch won the Nobel Prize in 1905, the citation was for his discovery of the tuberculosis bacillus, which was the complete demonstration of his method. Cholera nearly fitted. To be precise, there were flaws in Koch's evidence and logic: despite his best efforts, he couldn't infect an animal with the bacterium. But that didn't matter to his political masters of Germany, who were willing to gamble that his discovery would be vindicated. On Koch's return to Berlin in May 1884, the kaiser decided to treat the scientific breakthrough as a national 'victory' and the bacteriologist as a war hero. The announcement of the official banquet to honour the members of the Calcutta expedition and its 'commander' Koch read: 'Just as thirteen years ago the German people celebrated a glorious victory against the hereditary enemy of our nation [i.e. France], so does German Science today celebrate a brilliant triumph over one of humanity's most menacing enemies . . . Cholera.'[94] This, as we noted at the very start of the chapter, was the medal that Koch treasured as his favourite honour.

The public announcement mentioned the war against France, a classic Clausewitzean war between European states. A subplot in that war had been Germany's mastery over microbes, in this case smallpox. Field Marshal Helmuth von Moltke, chief of staff of the Prussian and then imperial German army, and an ardent admirer of Clausewitz, ensured that his army was ahead of its rivals in methodically interrogating medical impediments to military effectiveness. Germany vaccinated its troops against smallpox, and the Franco-Prussian war of 1870 was won in the clinic as well as on the battlefield. Afterwards, the Prussian Statistical Office scrupulously compiled the data. The two armies each deployed 150,000 troops. Among the unvaccinated French soldiers, 25,077 died of smallpox; in the vaccinated German ranks, just 297.[95] Smallpox didn't win the war – three times as many French soldiers died in combat – but it was an impressive reduction in the frictions enumerated by Clausewitz. The French recognized this too, and the shock of the defeat energized a state commitment to science, which included elevating Pasteur to a national icon. The two nations became scientific rivals as well as political ones.

Even more compelling, however, was the way the military imagery fitted with ambitions for colonial conquest. When the kaiser fêted Koch, the staff at the palace were busy preparing for his grand imperial conference, a far bigger and more lavish event. Victorian-era adventurers had been escorted by African guides to places previously unknown to Europeans, where they planted their flags, and named mountains and lakes after their own monarchs, or sometimes themselves. Europe's leaders convened in Berlin in October 1884 to draw Europe's lines on Africa's map, delineating, naming, and taking possession of territories that they had never seen. This was the 'scramble for Africa', and the rivalry was a combination of prestige (colouring the largest land areas English pink or French blue) and grabbing raw materials for the industrial age. Belgium's King Leopold took personal authority over the Congo and exploited its people and rubber trees with casual but surpassing cruelty. Germany staked its claims in east, west, and southern Africa, and Queen Victoria added to them when she gave Mount Kilimanjaro to her nephew Wilhelm as a birthday gift two years later.

In the popular culture of the era, microbiologists were explorers too, and could stake their claims in the new landscape revealed by the microscope. The first gift of naming went to the pioneers themselves. In his early career, Koch had taken the then-standard approach of naming his discoveries in line with the emergent scientific taxonomy – *Bacillus anthracis*, *Mycobacterium tuberculosis*, and *Vibrio cholerae*. But that practice was changing, and naming was becoming nationalistic and competitive. Pasteur was the world leader in bacteriology and a French hero; Germany was determined to catch up. The bigger point is that for the readers of newspapers and magazines, the very fact that these microbes were being described and named meant that they could be mastered and controlled. Microbiologists were true explorers of a new world of new kinds of organisms which behaved in strange ways that sometimes had intuitive parallels with everyday phenomena (such as yeast in breadmaking, or insect colonies) and sometimes didn't. Scientists needed vocabulary and imagery to explain these, and for obvious reasons they didn't want to invoke the names of faeries and goblins. So, they invoked bugs, dirt, parasites, and invaders. Hostility to these things was shared by all sides in the controversies of the time.

Koch, however, began to adopt distinctively martial language. He wasn't the first physician to use this kind of imagery. Traditional Chinese medicine from the 2nd century BCE uses metaphors of fighting an invasion. In the 18th century, the Chinese physician-scholar Xu Dauchun compared the physician to a general, though within the Chinese theorizing of warmaking, which is strikingly different to the European one.[96] Koch was probably unaware of these. However, he would certainly have known the writing of the 17th-century English physician Thomas Sydenham: 'A murderous array of disease has to be fought against, and the battle is not for the sluggard.'[97] But whereas Sydenham was a dissenting puritan who had fought against his king in the English civil war, and neither asked for nor received royal patronage,[98] Koch was a decorated officer in imperial service. In 1888 he said:

Even in peacetime [infections] slink about and sap the strength of armies, but when the torch of war is lit, they creep out of their hiding places, rear their heads to tremendous heights and destroy everything in their path. Proud armies have often been decimated, even destroyed by epidemics; wars, and with them the fate of nations, have been decided by them.[99]

Koch went further. Not only were bacilli 'public enemies' and cholera an invisible alien lurking in the jungles of Bengal ready to attack civilization, but he depicted the human body as a battlefield in which physicians and bacteria contest for control.[100] And, for the first time, there emerged the idea that science could declare war on disease, and win. Thus was conceived military-medical modernity.

The Train from Berlin

Cholera's fifth pandemic lasted from 1881 to 1896. The average death toll in India over the years 1892–6 was 443,890.[101] There were 200,000 dead in Russia.[102] It again devastated the Hajj, killing 33,000 pilgrims out of 200,000 in 1893.[103] But its final stand in Europe was in Hamburg, Germany's most cosmopolitan city. This was also the field test of the war on the disease.

Cholera arrived in Hamburg in August, almost certainly by train with Jewish migrant artisans, expelled from Moscow by Tsar Alexander III. The forced emigrants gathered their possessions and moved westwards through Poland to Germany, hoping to buy passage to New York. Germany had sanitary inspections on its eastern frontier, where passengers had to change trains because the railway gauges were different each side of the border, but cholera slipped through, as it was wont to do.

On the night of 14–15 August 1892, a doctor in the small town of Altona, just downstream from Hamburg outside the city limits, was called to see a building worker taken violently ill in the early hours of the morning with spasms of vomiting and diarrhoea. Dr Hugo Simon immediately diagnosed Asiatic cholera. However, his superior, Medical Officer Dr Wallichs, refused to accept this. The two had fallen out over their opposing political opinions, which had spilled over into a dispute over membership of the Hamburg Doctors' Club. Simon followed his superior's orders and his note on cause of death didn't mention cholera.[104] While most authoritarian centralizers were believers in germ theory and liberals were anti-contagionists, in this particular case, the two doctors' alignments were the converse: Wallichs had opposed Simon for his anti-Prussian sentiments. Within a few hours, their personal drama was no longer relevant. The outbreak and its politics were accelerating under their own momentum and shaping the denouement of Europe's epic fight against epidemic disease.

Cholera raged in Hamburg, its numbers following the exponential logic of an unconstrained microbial march through a population. From 16 to 23 August, the daily count of cholera cases was: 2; 4; 12; 31; 66; 113; 249; 338. On 27 August, 1,024 cases and 414 deaths were reported. But Hamburg's medical staff did nothing. Worse, they assured the captain of the steamship *Moravia* that it could sail for New York with its 385 passengers and a clean bill of health. Mark Twain was arriving just as it departed, and wrote about a city in denial, his wit muffled by his dismay. He complained that the city newspapers barely mentioned the epidemic, so that the mortality could only be guessed from the death notices posted by private citizens, and wrote, 'I know now that nothing that can happen in this world can stir the German daily out of its eternal lethargy. When the Last Day comes it will note the destruction of the world in a three-line paragraph and turn over and go to sleep again.'[105]

Hamburg's epidemic wasn't just a disaster, it was a scandal. The deaths of 10,000 citizens of Hamburg (out of a population of 330,000) were entirely preventable. The immediate culprit was *Vibrio cholerae* in the water. But the Hamburg Senate shares the blame. Despite the centralizing ambitions of the Prussian state, and the uniform colour of its territories on the political map of Europe, the administration of Germany was not yet unified. Slowly, standardized government was being applied across the patchwork quilt that had been the principalities, city-states, and episcopal estates of the former Holy Roman Empire. Among these, the civic republic of Hamburg was the outstanding exemplar of liberal self-government, a standing challenge to Prussian military centralism. Germany's second-largest city and its richest port, Hamburg still retained the legacy of self-government from its membership of the Hanseatic League. The city was run by its own senate and zealously guarded its powers to make independent policy decisions, especially in matters of trade. Indeed Hamburg was the most 'English' city in Germany, governed by an assembly of its citizens: by its constitution, a small and privileged group of property owners; by its social history, an oligarchy of traders and lawyers. Those citizens disliked and distrusted the military-bureaucratic Prussian ways of state. They believed in small government, balancing the books, and individual responsibility for health and well-being. Spending their tax money on a water filtration plant looked to be an extravagance that threatened both the fiscal health of the city-state and the ethic by which it had prospered. Although they had agreed to undertake this project, the construction was progressing without any urgency.

Crucially for the story of cholera, the senate appointed the city-state's medical officers – and chose them based on which school of thought they followed regarding infectious diseases. The school they favoured was Pettenkofer's, who had headed the cholera commission in Berlin until usurped – as he saw it – by Koch.[106] Hamburg just carried on faithfully following the policies that the Prussian government had advocated before Koch abruptly reversed them. Pettenkofer didn't concede gracefully and seems to have even hardened his antipathy to the waterborne hypothesis. Perhaps he was also persuaded by the echo chamber of his loyal students and his commercial fan club, who had other reasons for expounding those views – like their English counterparts earlier in the century, they considered quarantine as much of an evil as the disease itself.

Hamburg's first and most calamitous error was repeatedly postponing the construction of filtration plants to treat the city's drinking-water supply, so that people were drinking water piped from the river Elbe to storage tanks and from there to their homes. As water levels dropped in the dry, hot summer of 1892, contaminants were washed by the tides and currents from riverside towns and from the barges that plied the waterway. The microbes were more concentrated in the dwindling water in the reservoirs. Filtering through sand efficiently removes *Vibrio cholerae*. Other cities did it. Hamburg didn't. The senators were selfish, perhaps, but they were also consistent in their individualistic dogma. Some of their actions were laudable: they didn't blame Jewish migrants for bringing cholera to the city and they didn't want to deploy soldiers to enforce a lockdown.

The next-biggest failing of Pettenkofer's disciples in Hamburg – especially chief medical officer Dr Johann Kraus – was their refusal to accept the cholera diagnoses and issue a cholera declaration during those crucial days in August when the rate of infection was doubling each day. Cholera can spread and multiply at an exponential rate. The delay of a day can make the difference between containing an outbreak and facing an epidemic.

Why did they not do this? Part of the explanation is the intellectual inflexibility of men of high standing. The other part is material interest. Seaport that Hamburg is, in the 1890s its economy, and the prosperity of its plutocrats, depended on keeping the harbour open and the ships moving. Goods were coming in from England and the United States. The larger part of Germany's exports were arriving by barge and train to be loaded onto ships destined for every continent, and the Hamburg–America line had regular sailings for New York, the decks packed with migrants seeking a better life on the far shore of the Atlantic. Four ships sailed while cholera raged unacknowledged in Hamburg; three of them carried people infected with cholera, of whom 76 died at sea and a further 44 at Swinburne and Hoffman Islands, from where on a clear day they could see the shiny new Statue of Liberty.[107]

Koch, 50 years old and at the height of his power, had moved into his new office in Berlin's Schumannstrasse, temporary home of the Royal Prussian Institute for Infectious Diseases, just seven weeks previously. He would have been aware that the epidemic warning lights were blinking red. As soon as he received the samples from Altona, he knew he had to go to Hamburg, though he didn't yet know how far the outbreak had proceeded. Following the same track as the cholera bacterium, Koch arrived at Hamburg railway station on the morning of 24 August.[108] With him on the train arrived not just his entourage but also a freight of imperial administrative capacity and martial metaphor. There was no official delegation at the station to meet the kaiser's consul. Koch had to make his own plans: his first stop was the city medical office, where he arrived at 9.00 a.m. Dr Kraus turned up only 30 minutes later, and had little information to impart, for he had done nothing other than sneer at the 'hyperactive behaviour' of his counterparts in other towns (such as Altona). Koch's next stop was the New General Hospital in Eppendorf, where the director, Dr Theodor Rumpf, was ready to greet him at the door. Koch asked straightaway if there were cholera cases to report, and Rumpf promptly gave him the figures, whereupon Koch remarked to his companion, 'The first man in Hamburg who's telling us the truth!'

After visiting the hospitals, disinfection centres, and barracks where the migrants from Russia were housed awaiting their ships, Koch toured the old, overcrowded, ramshackle Alley Quarters in the city centre. By this time, he was becoming aware that hundreds were already dead. 'I felt as if I was walking across a battlefield,' he said. Amid these unsanitary streets, courtyards, and canals, he was shocked: 'In no other city have I come across such unhealthy dwellings, such plague spots, such breeding places of infection.' His audience knew they were listening to a man who had scoured the Alexandria and Calcutta hospitals in his search for the bacterial culprit. In the alleys, he made a remark that became an infamous condemnation of Germany's most cosmopolitan city: 'Gentlemen,' he said, 'I forget that I am in Europe.'[109]

On the kaiser's authority, Koch took command of Hamburg's health administration. He brought in his own men to replace the senate's appointees, purging the medical office of Pettenkofer's loyalists. He demanded and got mass disinfection and systematic patient isolation. He insisted that all drinking water be boiled and he hastened the completion of the water filtration plant. It was more than a defeat for the old guard, it was a humiliation.

The Hamburg epidemic waned by the end of September. Despite the horrible death toll, Pettenkofer still fought a rearguard action during the official investigation into the outbreak. The old man conceded that the *Vibrio cholerae* was the (x) of the disease, but insisted that the (z) also needed to be explained. He posed the questions left unanswered: why were some locations spared while others were stricken? He reprised his argument from eight years earlier that because none of Koch's attempts to infect guinea pigs, cattle, fowl, and rabbits with the bacillus had succeeded, he hadn't actually met his own standard of proof. The other experimental strategy Koch could have taken was the courageous (perhaps foolhardy) practice of testing his theory on himself.[110] Pettenkofer rose to this challenge in what became one of the most famous self-experiments of all time. He threw down the gauntlet to Koch: he would drink a solution containing the cholera *Vibrio* and see what happened. If the bacillus was indeed the sole cause of the disease, he argued, he would surely contract it. Pettenkofer requested a sample of a solution containing the *Vibrio*, and Koch's assistants duly sent one. He drank it on 7 October, in his own words, ready to 'sacrifice both life and health for the higher ideals'. Had he been wrong, he wrote: 'I would have looked Death quietly in the eye for mine would have been no foolish or cowardly suicide; I would have died in the service of science like a soldier in the field of honor.'[111] He neutralized his stomach acids by drinking bicarbonate of soda before swallowing the broth

– truly the act of a brave man. He got sick with severe diar-rhoea, recording the grotesque symptoms in his diary. After a very disagreeable week, however, Pettenkofer recovered, concluding that his theory had been vindicated: germ (x) on its own wasn't enough.[112] In the history of medicine, this is recorded as a courageous oddity, the futile heroism of the defeated. It was a good individual performance, but Koch's was much grander.

Koch had won. The naysayers' defences collapsed; the conqueror imposed his will. The unresolved medical and epidemiological controversies of the day became only minor waystations on the iron railway of progress, through which the express train of medical science could rush with only a blast of a whistle to warn loiterers to get out of its way. Instead of infectious disease being understood as the co-production of the x, y, and z of pathogens, the environment, and the human host, they came to be seen as solely the work of the germ. Henceforth, germs and diseases were defined by Koch's methods, just as imperial territories were delineated by exploration and cartography, and subject peoples were defined by how they were conquered and administered. It was also a triumph for Germany over its rivals France and Britain, and authoritarian Berlin had proved its case over lib-eral Hamburg.

With victory came the right to write history. The scien-tific, political, and personal rivalries between contagionists and anti-contagionists weren't of interest to the public. What mattered was the validation of the radical new story for public health. This was the 'war on disease' narrative, in which science and military-style public health would fight and conquer an invisible enemy. It was still a draft with a clunky plotline, but it is a fable whose basics didn't change over the following 130 years.

3

Metamorphosis: Influenza

Franz Kafka contracted influenza in October 1918. He was living in Prague as a subject of the Austro-Hungarian empire, ruled by the Habsburgs, heirs to the Holy Roman Empire. He fell desperately ill while a long-awaited revolution was played out in the streets below his family's apartment and he rose from his sickbed five weeks later as František Kafka, citizen of the newly declared Republic of Czechoslovakia. In his biographer's words, it was 'scary and strange', or in an alternative translation, 'eerie but a bit comical'.[1]

The oddities go deeper, some of them strangely suitable for the author of a book with a plotline in which the protagonist is overnight transformed into a giant insect[2] – though the more accurate representation would be a chimera of an insect with the brain of a human being. The influenza pandemic 'slipped to the third page of many daily newspapers'.[3] The empire was collapsing; armies were no longer fighting; the principle that subjects should obey their rulers suddenly made no sense and people no longer had any fear of the soldiers deployed in the streets. On the first day of Kafka's illness, troops cordoned off the Altstädter Ring, where his family apartment was located. The next day they melted away and the protesters took over the streets, swarming towards Wenceslas Square, where, by force of numbers, they willed a new revolutionary order into being. Kafka's biographer, Reiner Stach, observes that 'just when there were finally good reasons to prohibit large gatherings, the public space had slipped out of government control. Demonstrations and national rallies had become hot spots where history was being made – and people were not covering their mouths with handkerchiefs.'[4] Kafka had long imagined this day; he had written about what the end of the war and the end of empire would mean for his own career as a writer. But as the political drama unfolded under his window, he was deep in a flu-induced fever, from which – already weakened by tuberculosis – he never fully recovered.

The Great Influenza of 1918–19 is the totemic pandemic of modern times. It is the biggest-ever mass mortality episode of the last two hundred years, regardless of what metric is used – total numbers or proportion of population. As historical demographers have become more skilled in their use of statistical methods, the estimates have crept up from 21 million dead at the time to today's best figure of somewhere between 60 million and 100 million.[5] This wide span of estimates is a commentary on influenza's disguise as an everyday ailment and its propensity to kill indirectly through increasing the lethality of other illnesses such as tuberculosis or heart disease. The toll is at least three times more than those killed in the Great War and commensurate with the combined total of deaths from violence and hunger during World War II.

Stranger still than Kafka's own story is the way in which the locomotive of world history metamorphosed – for an instant – from the god of war into the tiniest quasi-living thing, an assortment of RNA that is the shapeshifting influenza virus. Writing the story of influenza demands Kafka's ability to see what is alien in the familiar and what is normal in the strange. The influenza pandemic is the deepest mystery in the history of disease. There's a virological mystery:

where did it come from and where did it go? And there's a historical mystery: why is the biggest episode of mass death since the Great Plague missing from the history books? As we explore the pandemic, we realize that there are other, more insightful ways of posing these questions.

The quarter-century after cholera struck Hamburg was the heroic age of microbial medicine. The popular plot for the influenza pandemic was therefore already written in advance: medical scientists would identify the invisible enemy, develop a cure or a vaccine, and in the meantime the authorities would apply, with military efficiency, methods of transmission control to contain the outbreak. But influenza didn't follow this script. Science didn't find a biomedical solution. It was, in the words of the scholar of literature Elizabeth Outka, a 'plotless tragedy'.[6]

The War before the War

At the beginning of the 20th century, political economists determined that conventional war between the great powers of the day was a 'great illusion' – to be exact, a great irrationality.[7] The real wars of the day were 'small wars' in which the European and American powers 'pacified' the last frontiers and tamed the last wildernesses. Colonizing the tropics was an operation to suppress tropical diseases as well as native peoples.

Germ theory provided the 'enemy' for the archetypal 'war on disease' script. The term 'magic bullet' was coined in 1909 by the German doctor Paul Ehrlich, credited with finding a cure for syphilis that would strike the pathogen without harming its human host. The bacteria causing different diseases – tuberculosis, cholera, plague, pneumonias – were being isolated by microbiologists and would in due course become eradicable. The other part of the script, reserved for those pathogens that could be studied but not directly observed, known at the time as 'filterable viruses',[8] was the possibility of campaigns to eradicate them. It seemed inevitable that every infectious disease would one day soon have its cure or vaccine.[9]

The foundational story of American disease control is the conquest of yellow fever. It's also the prequel to influenza, because this was how Americans expected the influenza epidemic script to play out. The hero is Major (later Colonel) Walter C. Reed, who is famous as the captain of a team of dedicated and selfless heroes who conducted courageous and clever disease-detective experiments, celebrated in magazines, paintings, novels, and school textbooks, as well as the scientific literature.[10] The nation's most prominent military hospital is named after Reed, reintroduced to Americans on each occasion the president needs medical treatment.

Yellow fever was endemic to Africa and was trafficked across the Atlantic on slave ships. From the 18th century, outbreaks of the disease devasted the southern cities of the United States, occasionally reaching as far north as New York. Philadelphia – then the capital city – was stricken by a particularly terrible epidemic in 1793. It was known as the 'American Plague'. In the revolutionary era, it also protected the United States because Napoleon's army in Santo Domingo was so depleted by the disease that he was unable to reinforce French forces in Louisiana, and later sold the territory. The United States enforced Mediterranean-style quarantine measures, but not always effectively. An epidemic in 1878 began in New Orleans and spread throughout the lower Mississippi Valley, affecting more than a hundred cities and towns. Overall, 120,000 people were infected and one in six of those died. The cause of the disease was a puzzle: its outbreaks were unpredictable; it spread as if by an invisible and odourless miasma but didn't seem to be directly contagious. It affected rich and poor alike and was indifferent to the quality of sanitation. For decades, the US Postal Service disinfected its mail deliveries, fearing that letters and parcels might be a means of transmission. And yellow fever was virulent. During the Spanish–American war, more American soldiers died from yellow fever, malaria, and other diseases than from combat.

Reed was a military physician. In 1900, shortly after the US army occupied Cuba, he arrived in Havana as the head of a team that included three younger doctors, James Carroll, Aristides Agramonte, and Jesse Lazear. His task was to identify the agent that caused yellow fever and find a way of extirpating the disease. He succeeded in the first, after which the US army corps of engineers accomplished the second. Thus was yellow fever beaten in Cuba, Panama, and the United States itself. The detective work was a series of controlled experiments in which volunteers were exposed to the suspected agents of infection, which included the body fluids and fomites (blankets, clothing, and cutlery) of yellow fever patients, and mosquitoes. In one trial, some volunteers lived in close proximity to individuals sick with the disease, exposed to any transmission that might occur through fomites or yellow fever's black vomit, but carefully protected from mosquito bites through screens. None fell sick. Others were exposed to carrier mosquitoes but protected from fomites and person-to-person contagion. They contracted the disease. The investigators were brave. They experimented on themselves, and one died.

After Reed had proved his case, Dr William Gorgas, the army chief health officer for Havana, implemented a rigorous campaign to eradicate mosquitoes from the city. Army teams ensured that every yellow fever patient was isolated behind a screen to prevent mosquitoes from feeding and picking up the virus. They fumigated every building and identified every well, cistern, pond, or other site of standing water where mosquitoes might breed, which was drained or covered with a film of oil. This succeeded beyond expectations and a year later no cases of yellow fever were reported in Havana. As a positive by-product, malaria deaths decreased as well. Gorgas then went on to repeat the feat in Panama, clearing the sanitary path for the construction of the canal. All this was done before the virus could actually be seen.

Reed wasn't the first: others had beaten him to his discovery. A handful of pioneers had suspected the mosquito and carried out experiments and observations. They were no less brave, nor less creative, and a compilation of their results would have been no less conclusive. But the anti-contagionist medical establishment ignored or dismissed them. Among them were Stubbins Ffirth, John Crawford, and Louis Beauperthuy.[11] Most systematic was Carlos Finlay, a Cuban physician whose systematic experiments prefigured Reed – and indeed, when Reed arrived in Havana, Finlay shared his findings and also his prized collection of mosquito larvae.[12]

The first phase of Reed's experimentation was shoddy and dangerous. Carroll – a sceptic of the mosquito theory – was deliberately inoculated and developed yellow fever. He recovered, though he suffered life-long complications. Lazear inoculated a young soldier who also came down with fever. Lazear himself was then bitten by the same mosquito,[13] developed fever, and died. Reed made himself absent at this particular time and he never experimented on himself – a fact over which hagiographies quietly skated.[14]

Medical self-experimentation is limited by the small number of experimenters, and so cannot provide statistically valid conclusions. Reed's second and third rounds were more systematic, using more than 40 volunteers, including soldiers and Spanish immigrants to the United States who signed up in part for the $100 bonus payment. According to one of those who enrolled, 'Volunteering to Dr Carroll for experimental yellow fever was, I can assure you, a cold-blooded business proposition. There were no heroics in it as far as I was concerned. . . . I suspected that I would probably get it spontaneously anyhow, so I decided I'd rather have it under favorable circumstances.'[15] Three died: two immigrants and the only female subject, a contract nurse with the recently formed Army Nurse (Female) Corps named Clara Louise Maass.[16] Her death caused outrage: her mother described it as 'little short of murder', and one of Reed's team refused to perform any more experimental inoculations. As a result, for the first time in the history of medical experiments, Reed introduced a process of informed consent for participants in trials.

The purpose of the campaign was to help the United States become a colonial power in Central America. As the construction of the Panama Canal neared completion, Gorgas told the graduating class of medical students at Johns Hopkins University, '[O]ur sanitary work at Panama will be remembered as the event which demonstrated to the white man that he could live in perfectly good health in the tropics; that from this period will be dated the beginning of the great white civilization in these regions.'[17] Among the clauses in the US–Panama treaty was a requirement that Panama comply with the United States' sanitary ordnances, or forfeit administration of the territories adjoining the canal zone. The suppression of yellow fever was a signal triumph that placed the United States alongside France and Germany in the vanguard of civilization's war on disease.

At this time, germ theory was transforming military medicine from remedial damage containment to systematic prevention. The last major European conflict of the age before microbial medicine was the Crimean War of 1853–6. It wasn't the worst case of contagions incapacitating armies, but it was one of the best documented. Journalists' reports and the letters of the volunteer nurse Florence Nightingale publicly exposed the shocking lack of care for the sick and wounded, while improved record keeping meant that sickness and death could be tabulated. Almost one-quarter of British and French soldiers died from disease, three times the number killed in battle or who died of wounds.[18] As many as two-thirds of the Russian soldiers became unfit for service or died from disease and exhaustion.[19] The American Civil War was comparable, with two-thirds of its 660,000 military fatalities caused by diseases, especially typhoid, pneumonia, malaria, and yellow fever.[20] Fifty years later, the major powers had almost completely eliminated camp fevers and ship diseases. The British army lagged behind, catching up only after the ravages of epidemics during the Boer War. There was a dark side to this progress. Suppression of typhus probably did more to make 20th-century warfare possible than any other single innovation.[21] The epidemiological limit on war-waging had been lifted, allowing far larger armies to be deployed in the field in conditions that would have been disease traps just a few years earlier. Military campaigns had always been limited in size and duration by infectious disease. No longer.

My purpose here is not to debunk the achievements of Reed and Gorgas but to make the point that those celebrated triumphs inscribed the narrative of the 'war on disease' into popular expectations. Certain pathogens follow logics that mean that they can be 'defeated' by these standardized methods. When influenza struck in 1918, Europeans and (especially) Americans were confident that medical science would prevail. Unfortunately, influenza wasn't susceptible to the technologies of the day.

Scientific medicine could also turn germs into weapons and remove the necessities of life – food, water, even air – from enemies. Military chemists developed poison gases. Military epidemiology and pest control extended to counter-insurgency, sometimes genocidally so: for example, the extirpation of the Herero in German South-West Africa between 1904 and 1907 by driving them into the desert and poisoning their water wells, or the British invention of the concentration camp and the barbed-wire fence during the Boer War. These horrors were well understood and humanitarians campaigned against them. Not appreciated at the time were the implications of creating a new artificial ecology for mass warfare – something, indeed, that is still not fully understood today. In suppressing every known microbial threat to a population of young men, the warring powers created a unique ecosystem that could have been specifically designed for the evolution of a new pathogen of surpassing virulence. Looking back a century later, we can see this as a kind of martial micro-Anthropocene, local and transient, but an ominous portent for what has followed.

The Jester

If the influenza virus is to be cast as a character, it should be a court jester, parodying the human protagonists and making their pretensions seem absurd and hubristic. In 1918, influenza mocked the 'war' on disease. It also compelled new thinking about microbes, because viruses are a different sort of protagonist to bacteria. Viruses are alive only insofar as they inhabit their hosts, and otherwise are inert configurations of machinery – more like puppets than living actors, except that *they* pull the strings. Moreover, influenza is an oddity among viruses, a shapeshifter by design. The jester is ever changing its costume, borrowing bits and pieces from a chaotic wardrobe. In fact it's less a unitary character and more like a swarm. But it is an agent of history nonetheless.

Infectious pathogens usually trade transmissibility off against virulence in the host – they are normally heavy on one and not on the other. The 1918 influenza was vicious on both counts. Despite a hundred years of research, there's a lot we don't know – and the more we learn, the less confident we are about what we think we know.[22]

Influenza has three key character traits that make it into our jester. The first is that the virus's replication is prone to error. Its clones dress hastily and appear in random new combinations of garments, and it doesn't much care. This is known as 'antigenic drift', which creates new subtypes. Second, should two of these viral subtypes meet, lodging in the same host cell, they can exchange entire segments of genetic material. They can swap shirts or shoes. This 'reassortment' can happen in any host, bird or mammal. It is known as 'antigenic shift'. Occasionally, the strain with the new garb commands the stage, and in the third trait it drives out all the others. This happens because (to mix metaphors) the immune system acts like certain police departments that make arrests on the basis of stereotypes, first rounding up those who fit a generic profile and only later chasing down the cannier culprits who escaped the first sweep.

Today it is possible to sequence the newly drifted and shifted genetics of each influenza strain and obtain a precise determination of how it is related to previous ones. However, the naming system of the 1950s has proven simple and reliable and remains in use.[23] This is a craftsman's nomenclature, based on the measurements needed in the workshop to categorize the strain and develop a vaccine. It's like a card index that categorizes the strain according to immune response tests. The classifications don't indicate much about transmissibility or virulence. But the naming system is much more than a quirk of the history of microbiological method. It's the basis for the agreed diagnostic technology that virologists use to determine whether or not a strain qualifies as 'new'.[24] Given that any sample of influenza virus isn't an identical genotype but a spread of genetic variants, deciding on what qualifies as a distinct disease entity isn't self-evident. Rather, it's a matter of consensus among a peer group of expert virologists. This isn't just an academic matter, because if a strain of influenza is 'new' it will – by definition – qualify as 'pandemic'. The technicalities of microbial measurement can have global repercussions. We will return to this in chapter 5.

Avian influenza virus has a reservoir in ducks, geese, gulls, and related waterfowl. It's endemic to these birds, a mild disease for them, indicating that it is likely to be an aeons-old mutual adaptation. Avian influenza often infects other species of birds, and the more distant the species, the more pathogenic it tends to become. It can also cross to mammals: pigs, dogs, horses, and, of course, humans. There is every reason to suppose that humans have been infected with influenza for as long as they have had some contact with waterfowl. Influenza epidemics, however, could occur only when human populations were large and interconnected. Epidemics are as old as the historical record, though the varied symptoms mean that they have not always been diagnosed as such. An epidemic described by Hippocrates in 412 BCE is widely believed to have been influenza. There were scores of epidemics between 1173 and 1875 in Europe, with 15 crossing continents.[25] One struck Africa and Europe in 1510 and another went global in 1580. Spain was in that century the nation with the furthest-reaching intercontinental trade, and its cities were hard hit. The name derives from the Spanish *influencia* and the common belief that it was spread by a malign alignment ('influence') of the planets. There is a certain insight in this name: influenza returns with a timing that suggests a hidden regularity that mathematicians might be able to unravel. An irregular drumbeat of epidemics continued, slowly increasing in tempo, as the changing ecologies of *Homo sapiens* and domesticated animals (chicken, pigs, and horses) and the connectedness of the world, through steamships, railways, and later air travel, made worldwide transmission feasible. The jester was dipping its hands into the lottery bag more often, and the pool of potential winnings was getting ever bigger. Or, to stick with our costume metaphor, the joker was rummaging in a bigger and more expensive wardrobe with the chance of running around more widely before being recognized and apprehended. There have been eight influenza pandemics[26] in modern times: 1831–2, 1848–9, 1889–91, 1918–19, 1928–9, 1957–8, 1968–9, and 2009–10. In seven of these cases, the pandemic disease wasn't more virulent than the usual seasonal malady – it just infected more people.[27] There is just one exception: the influenza pandemic of 1918–19, which infected more people *and* was also far more lethal.

How It Began

One day in 1918, somewhere in the world, the jester's lottery drew a lethal sequence of numbers. It probably required two draws: one strain became well adapted to ease of transmission while another became dressed in uniquely fatal garb, and the two met. The progeny was supremely well aligned for velocity of transmission, speed of disease progression to lethality, and selecting young adults, especially men.[28] It raced around the world and then vanished. No subsequent strain has come close to matching its power. The pandemics of 1928–9, 1957–8, and 1968–9 each killed more than a million people, but the special qualities of the 1918 virus remained a terrifying puzzle.

When the Great War began in 1914, Britain's chief medical officer addressed the troops, advising them that they needed to defend against bacilli as well as bullets, and that they should be alert towards but unafraid of the former.[29] His German counterparts commissioned a systematic study of the 'war pestilences' that would imperil the troops in every territory through which they advanced.[30] Chief among their fears was typhus, which has a good claim for having decided the outcomes of the Balkan front in 1914–15 and the Eastern Front in 1916–17 when it selectively ravaged the armies of the belligerents at crucial moments,[31] though it was well controlled on the Western Front. When the United States entered the war in 1917, US Surgeon General William Gorgas – promoted to that position on account of his record in the yellow fever campaigns – promised that the campaign against Germany would be the first in which fewer soldiers died of disease than in combat. Speaking to *American Magazine* in March 1918, he stated: 'At this stage of the war many commanders report that their soldiers are in better health, even in the trenches, than our civilian population is here at home. There are fewer colds on the battle line in France than there are on Broadway. And the same thing is true of more serious troubles.'[32] Allowing for the fact that he was on a recruitment drive – speaking to the mothers of recruits, and therefore putting the best possible gloss on the dangers facing their sons – Gorgas described impressive advances in controlling diseases and treating injuries. He also provided discreetly worded advice on how best to handle soldiers' propensity to catch venereal diseases.

Medical officers at the time pointed to the ways in which the war and the mobilization for war, notably transatlantic troop transports and supply ships, facilitated the faster and wider spread of the virus.[33] The theorist of viral evolution Paul Ewald makes a stronger case that it wasn't just coincidence that the deadly strain of influenza emerged at this time: 'The possible effects of war on the *evolution* of pathogen characteristics have been overlooked.'[34] Specifically, the Western Front was an ecology in which the virus no longer faced a trade-off between transmissibility and virulence. Ewald argues as follows.[35] Most infectious pathogens are transmitted when the host is mobile. A person who has mild symptoms and is moving around will infect more people than someone who is immobile with severe symptoms. This is the rationale for mobility restrictions to contain infections like influenza that spread easily. It's also why diseases that are most infectious in the period before they produce symptoms are most likely to spread. At the other end of the spectrum, pathogens that have evolved in hospital settings are most transmissible when they cause severe symptoms, because it's those symptoms that keep patients in that special environment. These are nosocomial infections spread by contact with physicians, nurses, other attendants, and the surfaces of hospital equipment and – *in extremis* – syringes and needles, helped along the way by neglect for routine hygiene. Cholera is a hybrid: it can be transmitted by the asymptomatic but its most efficient spread happens when the patient is sick with gross symptoms. In the middle are vector-borne illnesses such as malaria and yellow fever. A patient with the symptoms of these diseases will be immobile and less likely to swat insects feeding upon his or her blood. Unless of course that patient is safely screened behind a bed net or is in a house with protective screens. There's evidence that widespread use of screens and nets not only reduces the incidence of mosquito-borne infections but also drives the pathogens to adapt to be less virulent.

The direction of the evolutionary argument should be clear. European military medics succeeded in organizing a war that was, for three years, astonishingly disease-free. Soldiers at the front line complained of trench foot and typhoid, and there was seasonal influenza and pneumonia in the winter. The trenches were infested with rats. But in comparison to previous wars, the rates of casualties from contagious diseases were very low. Industrial war was also a relentless choreography of circulating millions of men from one overcrowded setting to the next. Ewald writes:

> The environmental conditions associated with the trench warfare of World War I could hardly have been more favorable for the evolution of extreme virulence of airborne pathogens like influenza. Soldiers in the trenches were grouped so closely that even immobile infecteds could transmit pathogens. When a soldier was too sick to fight, he was typically removed from his trenchmates. But by that time trenchmates often would have been infected because rates of shedding are highest at the onset of illness, which typically occurs two to three days after exposure. The sick individuals were generally moved between a succession of crowded rooms by a succession of crowded vehicles. Severely ill soldiers were transported along with the wounded to field hospitals, where they were usually laid on blanket-covered straw inside tents.[36]

The organization of transmission was quickly recognized at the time. Front-line troops were rotated every two weeks. Among many such observations, the historian Carol Byerly cites one medical officer writing: '[T]he railway journey with the men crowded into box cars had considerable influence in the increase of the infection in all companies.'[37] Packing American troops into overcrowded ships for transport across the Atlantic became a scandal among the small circle of military physicians and generals who were permitted to know (of which more below). After the war, influenza was added to the ranks of 'war diseases' and military physicians feared that it would accompany future mass mobilization.[38] The key point here is that the massive, coordinated, routinized, sustained confinement and rotation of young men, including a consistent pattern of exposing the uninfected to the infected, created a unique ecology in which an airborne pathogen could become as virulent as a nosocomial infection. The much-noted and puzzling anomaly that the 1918 influenza selectively struck young men is also explained: the virus adapted in precisely this demographic. And the rapid selection for milder strains after the end of the war is also explained.

The central element in Ewald's ecological hypothesis is viral evolution within the human population. Other aspects of the Western Front could also be relevant. There were increased risks of zoonotic transmission from the millions of military horses and mules, nearby farms with pigs, ducks, and geese, and nearby wetlands where migrating birds transited. The French army brought colonial troops from South-east Asia, a known reservoir of influenza, and there was an outbreak of what was called 'Annamite pneumonia' among Cambodian troops in April 2018. Anton Erkeka, who has chased down every possible clue looking for antecedents of the pandemic influenza, finds this intriguing, and writes, '[T]he spectacular virulence of the autumn 1918 epidemic wave could well have been contributed to by the recombination in Europe of viruses of Chinese and Indochinese origin.'[39] The impact of the 24 types of chemical weapons used in the war, some of which had mutagenic properties, is another potential contributory factor.[40]

The hypothesis that the 1918 influenza evolved in the trenches is supported by the observations of army physicians. This line of investigation has been most thoroughly pursued by John Oxford, who found that outbreaks of severe respiratory infections occurred at the British army camp at Étaples in northern France in 1916, which had high mortality (40 per cent) but very little person-to-person spread.[41] One doctor wrote in 1918: 'We emphasize our view that in essentials, the influenza pneumococcal purulent bronchitis that we and others described in 1916 and 1917 is fundamentally the same condition as the influenza pneumonia of this present 1918 pandemic.'[42]

The 1916 strain of influenza – if it was such – was hard to transmit, however, and either died away or lingered, causing just a few cases. However, the very fact that it had emerged showed how a virus could evolve in those conditions. That strain, or a similar one that emerged later, may have swapped its genes with another subtype, such as a highly transmissible strain documented in Kansas, which appears to have spread from west to east. Combining the contemporary clinical records, the ecological argument, and recent reconstruction of viral genetic subtypes, Oxford has proposed that the relatively minor genetic mutations needed could have occurred as the 1916 virus 'exchanged high lethality for a higher level of infectiousness as it moved in a grand circle from Étaples to the United States and back, in the bodies of the men of General Pershing's Expeditionary Force'.[43] Oxford's hypothesis is unproven but illustrates what we now know to be a feasible evolutionary pathway.

That evolutionary step might have taken place in the German trenches, where influenza cases were reported in April 1918.[44] The earliest evidence of something truly out of the ordinary was exceptionally virulent influenza among soldiers in June, as Germany massed troops for its final offensive on the Western Front. General Erich von Ludendorff redeployed millions of reinforcements from the Eastern Front, where the revolutionary government in Russia had agreed to peace terms. He was rushing to strike a fatal blow on the British and French lines before the American troops arrived *en masse*. In war-fighting, as in epidemic control, timing is everything. Just as the concentration of German troops and armour reached its peak, influenza mortality rates shot up like a rocket. A graph published by the German Bureau of Sanitation shows influenza deaths in the army during the war. It has seasonal waves peaking each late winter, and in

June 1918 the line literally goes off the charts.[45] From August 1917 until May 1918, mortality from influenza among the troops was between 3 and 4 per cent of the caseload, about where it had been since the beginning of the war. In June, 135,002 soldiers contracted influenza on the Western Front, with a case-mortality rate of 35 per cent. In July, 374,000 soldiers on the Western Front fell sick and the mortality rate also went off the scale, passing 100 per cent – which must reflect a time-lag between the wave of infections peaking even while the wave of deaths was still increasing.

The epidemic curve for German troops in the Balkans and on the Eastern Front followed the same pattern one month later. On the Allied side, the exponential increase of the virulent summer strain followed six weeks behind. A doctor with the American Expeditionary Force in France, Jefferson Kean, recorded in his diary on 17 August, 'Influenza increasing and becoming more fatal.'[46] Three weeks afterwards, it was recorded in Massachusetts; it was brought to Philadelphia on a British ship; a month later it was in Freetown, Sierra Leone.

There are two other origin theories, each based on outbreaks that started earlier in the year. One begins with southern China, the usual suspect for avian flu – and if one searches for outbreaks of influenza there, they are always to be found. It is possible that influenza travelled with Chinese workers recruited to fill the demand for labour in Britain and France. These labourers were shipped to Vancouver, British Columbia, where they reportedly suffered an influenza outbreak, and then travelled by train to the east coast of Canada before sailing to Europe.[47] The other widely cited claim to a place of origin is Haskell County, Kansas, site of a well-documented outbreak in the spring of 1918 that spread to two of the main centres at which army recruits were congregating, namely Camp Funston (Kansas) and Camp Ogleforth (Georgia).[48] Neither explanation is complete: they don't account for how regular influenza became the uniquely virulent pandemic variant. The wide acceptance of the Kansas origin tells us more about who tells the influenza story and why: most books and articles are written by Americans drawing on high-quality medical records. Historians of epidemics also like it because it's an intriguing inversion of the standard 'out there' origins script – in the words of John Barry, the leading historian of America's pandemic, investigators 'must look everywhere' for new viruses.[49]

Ewald's critics said his was an unproven hypothesis. By that logic, all evolutionary arguments are 'unproven' in the sense that they cannot be observed in the laboratory or rerun as controlled experiments. Shifting a scientific paradigm is never just about 'proof': it's also about a narrative that convinces and a scientific argument that gains authority. The evolutionary-ecological storyline doesn't fit the disease detective plotline, which is concerned with finding a single, identifiable pathogenic culprit to convict. Compare the two approaches to an explanation. The mainstream biomedical virologist focuses on the jackpot winning numbers. The ecologist asks what determines the odds, which means looking at how the casino is organized. It is the *only* explanation other than a vanishingly remote roll of the mutational dice that makes sense.

Influenza inverted the 'war on disease' script. In making it possible to wage mass war, military medicine made possible the emergence of this unique pathogen. In the triumph of modernity lay a danger beyond our capacity to anticipate, even to measure.[50] According to evolutionary viral logic, the Great Influenza was manufactured in the Great War, and was not just a fellow traveller.

'Warriors'

A well-documented outbreak of the uniquely virulent form of influenza struck the newly built army camp of Fort Devens, just outside Boston, Massachusetts, on 8 September 1918. The journal entries and letters of physicians at the camp – the biggest and most modern in America with the best medical facilities – show how physicians who had been schooled in the gruesome realities of war could still be shocked.[51] Young men marched in one day and overnight they became helpless wretches lying in their own filth, scarcely able to breathe, and by the following day their bodies were stacked like cords of wood in the morgue. One account, discovered in a trunk in Detroit 30 years afterwards, was later published in the *British Medical Journal*.[52] It is a letter written by Dr Roy Grist, an army doctor assigned to Fort Devens. He wrote:

These men start with what appears to be an ordinary attack of LaGrippe or Influenza, and when brought to the Hosp. they very rapidly develop the most vicious type of Pneumonia that has ever been seen. Two hours after admission they have the Mahogany spots over the cheekbones, and a few hours later you can begin to see the Cyanosis extending from their ears and spreading all over the face, until it is hard to distinguish the colored men from the white. It is only a matter of a few hours then until death comes, and it is simply a struggle for air until they suffocate.

Doctors compared its impact only to the poison gases used at the Western Front; men choking, literally drowning in the fluid released into their lungs. Later in his letter, Roy continues:

[W]e used to go down to the morgue (which is just back of my ward) and look at the boys laid out in long rows. It beats any sight they ever had in France after a battle. An extra long barracks has been vacated for the use of the Morgue, and it would make any man sit up and take notice to walk down the long lines of dead soldiers all dressed and laid out in double rows.

This grisly parody of a parade foreshadowed the ranked crosses in war cemeteries. The metronome of death continued in Devens and other camps, and on the troopships transporting soldiers from the ports on the east coast to France. That roll-call had quickened two months earlier in the German army. The virus had already helped halt the German summer offensive. Ludendorff wrote, 'Our army had suffered. Influenza was rampant, and the army group of Crown Prince Rupprecht was particularly afflicted. It was a grievous business having to listen every morning to the chiefs of staffs' recital of the number of influenza cases, and their complaints about the weakness of their troops.'[53] Barry notes caustically that 'Ludendorff was not one to accept blame when he could place it elsewhere.'[54] All the armies suffered, though incomplete records among the German, British, and French don't allow for a comprehensive comparison.[55] Of the 4 million men in the American Expeditionary Force, more than 1 million fell ill.[56] If Ludendorff was ready to blame his defeat on influenza, the Allies wanted to claim the victory for themselves, not for the virus. Although they had been puzzled by the strange lull in the German offensive in July, Allied explanations for their military success don't give much credit to influenza. To this day, the consensus view is that all armies suffered more or less equally, so that 'influenza had a profound impact on both the military apparatus and the individual soldier, but presumably less on the course of the war.'[57] This even-handedness doesn't take into account the importance of timing in war. Virulent influenza immobilized the German forces first – in June and July, when they had the initiative – and hampered the Allies in September and October, when the tide of battle had already turned. Possibly, the pathogen decided the encounter and the generals only mopped up afterwards.

Such is the grip of the 'war on disease' script that in his authoritative book *The Great Influenza*, John Barry titled the first section 'The Warriors', meaning the doctors and scientists racing to battle the disease.[58] He did not mean it ironically – he just didn't have another vocabulary to hand to commend the exemplary courage and dedication with which they, along with nurses and other health workers, treated the sick. Barry writes: 'Physicians, nurses, scientists did their jobs, and the virus killed them, killed them in such numbers that each week JAMA [*Journal of the American Medical Association*] was filled with literally page after page after page of nothing but brief obituaries in tiny compressed type. Hundreds of doctors dying. Hundreds.'[59] He documents the efforts of a small band of scientists to determine the cause of the disease, to find therapies, and to develop a vaccine. They are heroic, but in a minor key. There are no epic triumphs of microbiology or epidemiology; there is no disease detective story fingering the villain. There were also no great battles of scientific doctrine or ego, no rivalries among the Great Powers to be the first to name and tame the scourge. Barry tells a good story, but his raw material is disappointment.

At the time, influenza's aetiology wasn't known. But every scientist assumed that it was eminently – and imminently – knowable. Some progress had been made during the previous pandemic of 1889–91. Richard Pfeiffer, one of Koch's protégés and an accomplished bacteriologist, identified a bacillus found in most influenza patients. He was among the first to make a compelling case that influenza was a specific disease rather than a cluster of symptoms (or syndrome). Pfeiffer's proof was incomplete, and others found an apparently identical bacillus in patients suffering from other diseases such as whooping cough, measles, and bronchitis. But such was Pfeiffer's reputation, the enthusiasm for attributing bacterial causes to infections, and the absence of a rival theory that in 1918 most doctors accepted his bacillus was the agent.[60] Based on this, vaccines were developed, manufactured, and administered when the first cases occurred.

America's leading medical researchers were clustered in Boston, Massachusetts, close to the Fort Devens outbreak, and the city was the first metropolis to suffer an epidemic. Despite enthusiastic early reports of success, it quickly became clear that vaccination didn't appear to work. No-one had done systematic vaccine trials at speed before, and the controversies that followed prompted the American Public

Health Association to develop standards and protocols to protect human subjects (in this case, navy volunteers). The end result was desultory. No vaccine passed the test. No microscopist could identify the pathogen. The most likely suspect, Pfeiffer's bacillus, turned out to be an opportunistic secondary infection. When Edwin Jordan published his exhaustive volume *Epidemic Influenza* in 1927, he could conclude only that influenza's 'cause was unknown, and its pathology was indefinite. It was uncertain whether there was acquired immunity for influenza, and, if there was, how long it lasted. Why pandemics occurred when they did and why they spared some places were also unknown.'[61] In short, the pandemic passed without the medical warriors vanquishing their foe, or even sizing it up properly. It was in fact a backhanded tribute to the scientific method and the unchallengeable dominance of the germ theory of disease that these failures were not reason to challenge the paradigm, only to look harder.

Neither was there a formula for containment, just a handful of *ad hoc* mitigation efforts. The one crucial step that the governments in Berlin, Paris, London, and Washington, DC, could have taken to contain the pandemic was to stop the war and the mobilization for war. Of course, they did no such thing. Even when leaders understood, they remained gripped by a rage of numbers, obsessed with the calculation that the country that put the largest number of men and machines into the meat grinder of the trenches would be the winner. This justified the troop trains heading to the frontlines in France and Belgium, the feverishly expanded camps, and the packed troopships from Boston, New York, and Philadelphia. It was as though witless or fatalistic statesmen had surrendered decision to the relentless logic of war while historical agency passed unacknowledged to a virus.[62]

A case of terrible overcrowding was on the USS *Leviathan*, a troopship with a capacity of 6,800, which was fitted out with bunks to cram in 11,000 men.[63] Seven hundred fell sick on the first day out of New York. Attempts to isolate the infected broke down because there was no way of enabling the healthy and sick to eat in separate mess halls. The decks were soon slippery with the vomit and blood of the ill. At first, the army kept scrupulous records of illness and death, but, as Barry writes,

> a week after leaving New York, the officer of the day was no longer bothering to note in the log 'died on board,' no longer bothering to identify the military organization to which the dead belonged, no longer bothering to note a cause of death; he was writing only a name and a time, two names at 2:00 a.m., another at 2:02 a.m., two more at 2:15 a.m., like that all through the night, every notation in the log now a simple recitation of mortality, into the morning a death at 7.56 a.m., at 8.10 a.m., another at 8.10 a.m., and at 8.25 a.m.[64]

Eighty were buried at sea and the *Leviathan* docked at Brest, France, with 70 unburied bodies. Fourteen men died before they could be disembarked and several hundred in hospitals on shore.[65] This was October: even had they been healthy, these soldiers were arriving too late for the war.

Wartime censorship also meant that no government admitted the scale of its epidemics, with the exception of neutral Spain, so that the newspaper reports from the country meant that the disease earned the misnomer 'Spanish flu'. President Woodrow Wilson never once mentioned influenza in public.[66] Some officials even encouraged the spread of fear and of the rumour that the disease had been deliberately spread by the Germans.[67]

America's epidemic in the fall of 1918 and spring of 1919 provides a grand and gruesome natural experiment in what works and doesn't work containing an airborne respiratory virus. There was no federal policy, and as infections spread, each city was left to adopt its own set of policies. Boston was first, caught by surprise. Every other city had some advance warning and each set of municipal and health officials made their own decisions as to what to do. They were literate in basic sanitation and infection prevention from previous campaigns against yellow fever, cholera, and tuberculosis,[68] and could also follow the news from cities already affected. Because of the high quality of demographic and health statistics, the diligence of epidemiologists, and the renewed interest in such 'non-pharmaceutical interventions' (NPIs) in the 2000s, we can track the outcomes of the great influenza containment experiments of 1918.

The tragic drama of Philadelphia's epidemic earned a special place in the rolls of public health infamy.[69] Although influenza had already struck Boston and New York, and it was clearly a matter of days before it arrived in Philadelphia, the city authorities insisted that they go ahead with its biggest-ever public gathering. This was a 'Liberty Loan parade' to raise funds for the war effort. The city was doing its patriotic duty, in studied obliviousness to public health warnings. About 200,000 people packed the city centre. The result was as feared: the outbreak followed within two days and killed 12,000 people. The epidemic curve in Philadelphia takes the shape of a tall spire, the steepest of any city in the nation. It also had almost the highest mortality of any major US city; only Pittsburgh in western Pennsylvania fared worse, and more died per capita than Boston, where there had been no time at all to prepare.

By comparison, the city authorities in St Louis, Missouri, acted quickly. Within two days of detecting its first cases among residents, the city closed schools, playgrounds, libraries, courtrooms, and even churches. Work shifts were staggered and streetcar ridership was strictly limited. Public gatherings of more than 20 people were banned. St Louis 'flattened the curve' in 1918. The mortality peaked later at a level just one-eighth of that in Philadelphia. However, social distancing measures were relaxed before the epidemic had passed, and the numbers of infections shot up again, so that school closures and bans on public gathering had to be reimposed.[70] St Louis's epidemic curve has a two-humped pattern characteristic of cities that eased their lockdowns too early. The early success wasn't the whole story, but it was still important. Excess mortality over the pandemic period for Philadelphia was 748 per 100,000 and for St Louis 358 per 100,000, just under half.[71] Almost the same story can be told for Denver, Colorado, another city that flattened the first curve but reopened too early. A key difference is that Denver didn't reimpose a ban on public gatherings and instead implemented isolation and quarantine measures to try to dampen the second peak.[72] Other cities and states adopted variants of these measures. Photos from the period invariably show people wearing face masks, which became the emblem of the pandemic. People had become familiar with surgical masks from pictures of war surgeons, and this was the first time they were used by ordinary people. Mask wearing was usually a personal choice, although some cities enforced face masks in public.

Unfortunately, as an article in the 5 July 1919 *Literary Digest* concisely summed up the challenge, influenza's spread 'was simple to understand, but difficult to control'.[73] Recent studies in historical epidemiology, led especially by Howard Markel, have compared NPIs, infections, and deaths in different cities. They have found no measure that stopped the virus completely. Indeed, no single measure by itself had a statistically significant effect in reducing infections. What the research found was that quick implementation of multiple NPIs at the same time reduced influenza transmission and deaths by as much as 50 per cent. The cities that implemented NPIs earlier had greater delays in reaching peak mortality, lower peak mortality rates, and lower total mortality.[74] However, when the measures were relaxed, there was a danger that infection rates would rebound.[75] Complete isolation was only possible for a handful of really tiny communities, such as small islands, closed institutions like sanatoriums which already had restrictions on entry and exit, and remote towns. The town of Gunnison in the Colorado mountains is the *cause célèbre*: it sealed all the roads in and out and stopped all travel until the epidemic had passed. Contemporary researchers have called this 'protective sequestration' and shown that it was effective – in fact the only single NPI that works completely.[76] For obvious reasons, it was very rare. To work, protective sequestration had to be implemented early and sustained for long enough until the final wave of the epidemic had passed.

Lessons like this could only be learned many decades later when the data were compiled and better computational capacities and statistical methods were available. In 1918, people could nonetheless absorb the main points: namely that it was worth trying but that one could hope only to reduce the odds in the lottery of infection, and sometimes not by much. Nancy Tomes writes of the 'the irony of public health commentaries on the pandemic: few believed that practicing the gospel of germs had worked to control the outbreak, yet they continued to promote its value.'[77] This is the containment version of the microbiological paradox, which is that although science largely failed to conquer influenza, its minor victories were those that counted in the reckoning, and its defeats were put down to not having tried hard enough. Tomes calls it an 'odd combination of futility and certainty'.[78] Public institutions had to do and say *something*, because doing nothing – or, still worse, sending messages that nothing could be done – was bad for morale.

More than eight decades later, as pandemic preparedness plans were drawn up in America and Europe, this 'odd combination' recurred.[79] None of the lessons learned were very consoling. While Markel and his team identified the measures that would provide the guidelines for pandemic influenza containment, others argued that the effectiveness of NPIs was too modest to warrant the high social and economic costs. Donald Henderson, veteran of the smallpox campaign from the 1970s, co-authored a paper that argued that lockdown wouldn't work: 'Historically, it has been all but impossible to prevent influenza from being imported into a country or political jurisdiction, and there has been little evidence that any particular disease mitigation measure has significantly slowed the spread of flu.'[80] He and his co-authors challenged the logic of lockdown and social distancing: '[W]e must ask whether any or all of the proposed measures are epidemiologically sound, logistically feasible, and politically viable.'[81] The US Centers for Disease Control and Prevention (CDC) weighed the evidence, the debate, and the options, and came out in favour of containment using NPIs.[82] There's a double paradox here. First, the very basics of the success of our society and economy are what make us susceptible to pandemic influenza, and if we are candid, it cannot be stopped, only mitigated. Second, public institutions must do *something*, even if it isn't likely to work, because that's what they do, and what people expect them to do. Or, to put it another way: where science fails, the 'war on disease' script fills in the blanks to assure us that science just hasn't succeeded quite yet.

In 1918, influenza was global. It may have killed as many as 100 million people around the world. Its histories have yet to be written fully. Let me draw on just one other country's experience in which Tomes's paradox can be seen from a different perspective: South Africa. The infection arrived on troopships in September and spread rapidly, albeit unpredictably, with some communities ravaged and others spared.[83] Over the following weeks, one in ten people perished in some districts. In Ciskei, '[N]o war, army action or police brutality; no government law or proclamation; no drought, famine, flood, insect plague and animal disease . . . wreaked as much human carnage as "Black October".'[84] The historian Terence Ranger wrote, 'In its novelty, its generality, its capriciousness, its immunity to treatment, the pandemic was bound to give rise to intense speculation and to challenges to established systems of medical thought and practice, not least those of the missions and the colonial administration.'[85] Over the previous two generations, epidemic lungsickness and rinderpest among cattle and smallpox among people had caused social convulsion. People had noticed that these diseases accompanied the colonizers, and in the case of influenza, the infection followed the railway lines and exploded in the townships and in some mining compounds (though not others), afflicting Europeans and migrant labourers, while people living in remoter villages were spared. Western medicine didn't offer a cure; indeed, to the contrary, anyone going to a hospital was likely to fall sick. Ranger writes,

> It might appear as a divine judgement on the system of industrialization and migrant labour and a divine revelation of the inadequacy of the orthodox medical regimes at the mission stations themselves. . . . As many administrators wryly observed, Africans stood a better chance of survival the further away they were from the centres of western biomedical provision. In the rural areas the mission stations and boarding schools were themselves the first seats of the disease and there were many deaths. This was certainly an epidemic which revealed the impotence of missionary biomedicine and gave powerful stimulus to alternative ideas of causation and healing.[86]

The earlier epidemics of empire had fanned creative reinterpretations of customary prophetic traditions, some of them foreseeing the imminent end of the world. Influenza arrived at a time when mission Christianity had become dominant, and it prompted a new prophetic tradition within African Christianity. Prophets, healers, and diviners who diverged too far from what was recognizably Christian and who threatened the colonial order were repressed and their leaders incarcerated as criminals or lunatics. The devastating caprices of influenza further nourished abiding scepticism about western medicine. In America, popular faith in public health required the authorities to say and do something, even if it wasn't going to work. For South Africans, the logic worked the other way: it made more sense for people to ignore, subvert, or resist the gospel of germs and the logic of alien governing institutions relentlessly doing their thing.

The pandemic strain ran through populations on both sides of the Atlantic, around the coast of Africa, to India, and (remarkably) on to China.[87] It even reached the Arctic, and, after a delay in which sequestration measures worked for a while, it landed in Australia and New Zealand after those countries lowered their guard. The pandemic ended in the spring of 1919 when the virus retired undefeated.

A Story That Could Not Be Told

There was a profound silence around the pandemic. For historians of calamity, this is not a surprise. Veterans of the Great War were famously reticent about telling their stories from the trenches. Most survivors of the Holocaust left it to their children and grandchildren to reconstruct their experiences. The Great Famine inflicted upon the Irish people in 1845–51 is comparable in its aching absence, shadowing everything but nowhere acknowledged, until six generations had passed. An investigation by the journalist David Segal turned up just two public memorials to the 1918–19 influenza, one in Barre, Vermont, and the other in Wellington, New Zealand.[88] This silence descended at once. It was everywhere: America, Europe, Asia, Africa. Shortly afterwards, an editorial in *The Times* of London reflected:

> So vast was the catastrophe and so ubiquitous its prevalence that our minds, surfeited with the horrors of war, refused to realize it. It came and went, a hurricane across the green fields of life, sweeping away our youth in hundreds of thousands and leaving it a toll of sickness and infirmity which will not be reckoned in this generation.[89]

Where historians, political scientists, and journalists fear to tread, poets and novelists will venture. Influenza appeared in pulp fiction,[90] but it has to be read between the lines of post-pandemic literature, as a spectral presence, everywhere and nowhere.[91] Academics studied adjacent issues, as if averting their eyes from a light too blinding to gaze at directly. In 1919, the Dutch historian Johan Huizinga published his pioneering study of the 14th and 15th centuries in Europe – the era of the great bubonic plague and its aftermath – opening with reflections on the violent tenor of life, the pervasive cult of death, and the unending round of raucous ceremonies that enveloped Europe in those centuries.

> Calamities and indigence were more afflicting than at present; it was more difficult to guard against them, and to find solace. Illness and health presented a more striking contrast; the cold and darkness of winter were more real evils. Honours and riches were relished with greater avidity and contrasted more vividly with surrounding misery.[92]

Huizinga barely mentioned the Black Death, and influenza not at all. Two years later, post-war and post-pandemic Europe and America seemed to be living up to his portrait. The American sociologist James Thompson made the same comparison:

> The turmoil of the world today serves to visualize for us what the state of Europe was in the middle of the fourteenth century far more distinctly than ever was perceived before. It is surprising to see how similar are the complaints then and now: economic chaos, social unrest, high prices, profiteering, depravation of morals, lack of production, industrial indolence, frenetic gaiety, wild expenditure, luxury, debauchery, social and religious hysteria, greed, avarice, maladministration and decay of manners.[93]

Thompson dwelt on the war. He never once mentioned influenza by name, only referring in passing to the toll of 'some millions' from 'starvation, privation, and disease'.[94] Reprising the exact same parallel in his seminal book *The Black Death*, published in 1969, Philip Ziegler also doesn't mention the Great Influenza, only the Great War.[95] Influenza was an odd but conspicuous gap in the histories of disease and society for half a century – a literature review would consist in a long catalogue of absences and passing mentions of its enigma.

For example, it barely registers in William McNeill's *Plagues and Peoples*,[96] the book that inspired many history students to write their theses on epidemics. The second edition of Alfred Crosby's pioneering book on influenza was given the revealing title *America's Forgotten Pandemic*.[97] Asked to account for the amnesia in a recent podcast interview, John Barry replied bluntly, 'I can't explain it.'[98]

Some voices from the epidemic weren't silent, they were deliberately silenced. One of the South African prophets mentioned by Ranger was a middle-aged illiterate Xhosa woman named Nontetha Nkwenkwe. She suffered a severe bout of influenza during which she had scary and strange visions demanding that her people redeem their sins as the world was coming to an end. On rising from her sick bed, she founded a millenarian resistance movement that mixed Xhosa beliefs and Christian symbols. The authorities consigned her to a lunatic asylum and an unmarked grave, an oblivion from which the historians Robert Edgar and Hilary Sapire rescued her memory and bones many years later. They see Nontetha's 'madness' as silenced resistance, and her 'apparently dead-end deluded imaginings' as 'eloquent commentary on the most common sources of discontent with African societies, as well as a haunting accompaniment to the many dreams of and cries for redemption and renewal outside the asylum walls'.[99] Unlettered poets and prophets such as Nontetha can be seen as the unacknowledged Kafkas of the colonized.

Modern historians are also uncomfortable with the idea that something as unpredictable and apparently random as infection might have decided the course of history. It challenges the premises of their discipline; it just doesn't fit the task of making history intelligible. Their debates spin around human agents, who cause events or solve riddles. It was only 80 years on that historians of both left and right began to articulate the sheer *stupidity* of the war. The radical historian Gabriel Kolko decries the 'myopia' and 'striking repetitive eccentricities and perverse obstinacy of countless important men' who led their countries into needless wars which brought ruin upon their societies – and upon themselves.[100] On the political right, Niall Ferguson – rarely sharp at discerning hubris in Europe's aristocrats or financiers – concludes his book on the war: 'The First World War was at once piteous, in the poet's sense, and "a pity". It was something worse than a tragedy, which is something we are taught by the theatre to regard as ultimately unavoidable. It was nothing less than the greatest *error* of modern history.'[101] The first drafts of the story of the Great War were being written even as the armies were still fighting. At the time, none of them candidly faced the war's meaninglessness. Even Hans Zinsser, sanitary officer for the US army and biographer of typhus, looked away. He had insisted that military strategy and combat tactics 'are only the terminal operations engaged in by those remnants of the armies which have survived the camp epidemics',[102] but couldn't contemplate what influenza meant for that thesis. Many of the approximately 80,000 books on that war published over the last 100 years are re-fighting the war on the printed page, with diktat over the storyline going to the victor. By contrast, a book on the pandemic must acknowledge the principal protagonist's lack of motive or reason. The 400 books on the influenza are few by comparison, and most of them were written in the last 25 years.[103]

The Great Influenza cannot be written as epic. Barry recounts a dozen dramas – painful, moving, occasionally heroic, but not adding up to an epic. His *The Great Influenza* is the go-to telling of America's pandemic (the rest of the world is marginal), and it includes episodes such as the preventable outbreak in Philadelphia in which the virtues of patriotism and public health clashed with one another. Barry conjures to life obstinate villains such as the bumbling US Surgeon General Robert Blue, contrasting them with the humble dedication of microbiologists and municipal officers, who showed civic steadfastness and quiet bravery. It would be tempting to take one or more of these as morality tales that can serve as microcosms of the politics of the pandemic.

All, however, are too small in scale and too limited in scope to match the toll. The scores of millions of deaths were tragedy in the everyday sense: loss without redemptive meaning. They did not make a tragedy in the sense of a drama in which the protagonists play out their virtues and contests, finally reaching a denouement.

The Great Influenza could not be written as the triumph of progress. Nancy Bristow argues that the influenza pandemic threatened to expose the fragility of America's optimism: 'The influenza pandemic was, simply put, the wrong narrative for its time and place. To remember the pandemic would have required Americans to accept a narrative of vulnerability and weakness that contradicted their fundamental understandings of themselves and their country's history.'[104] America did not want to question its faith in the mastery of the natural world and its exceptional place in the political world. Therefore, people still believed in medical science, despite its biggest ever failure.

They had good reason to believe. Medical progress in the half-century that followed the pandemic was as impressive as in the previous decades. It was testament to the experimental method that by the mid-1920s much was known about the as-yet-unobserved viruses, and the virologist Thomas Milton Rivers was able to conclude, correctly, that they are obligate parasites that require living cells to reproduce. Only with the invention of the electron microscope in 1931 could viruses be directly studied. A spate of virological breakthroughs followed. A team in London isolated the influenza virus in 1933. The first influenza vaccines were developed in the 1950s, and the disease was reduced to a familiar seasonal ailment, often little worse than a bad cold. Progress in controlling other diseases was rapid. Tuberculosis and syphilis were brought under control. Typhus and plague were all but eliminated as threats to public health. In the 1950s, the WHO launched a campaign (modelled on the Gorgas yellow fever programmes) to eradicate malaria: it ultimately failed but made enormous progress nonetheless. A campaign against polio

was much more successful. The WHO achieved the greatest triumph of international medicine: the eradication of
smallpox in 1977. The US army, which had been terrified
that influenza might return with World War II and set up a
Board for the Investigation of Influenza and Other Epidemic
Diseases, scaled back its worries and abolished the successor institution, the Armed Forces Epidemiological Board, in
1971.[105] At that time, the US Surgeon General Dr William
Stewart was widely believed to have said, 'It is time to close
the book on infectious diseases, and declare the war against
pestilence won.'[106] It seems he never actually said it – but
it's the sort of thing that public health leaders were ready to
believe at the time.

The biography of pandemic influenza was the greatest
unsolved disease detective story of the 20th century, closely
followed by the mystery of where it went. In the spring of
1919, the jester played its last trick – or at least its last trick
in this act – and disappeared off-stage. Ten years later, it
returned, but it was less severe. When vaccines were developed, they weren't fully effective – a new one had to be
developed every year for the dominant strain. The detec-
tives' quest shifted. They weren't looking for a live suspect
hidden away somewhere but trying to work out what made
that historic culprit so lethal. To do that they needed to find
an intact specimen. For a small band of pathogen sleuths,
this became an obsessive quest – one in which they ultimately succeeded.

This passage in the annals of medical research could
have been copied from the heroic age of microbiology. It
involved two intrepid Arctic expeditions by a virus hunter-
turned-archaeologist, and the reconstruction of history's
potentially most lethal pathogen in a laboratory – a venture
as potentially hazardous as the Manhattan Project to build
the first atomic bomb. The story begins in 1951 when a
young Swedish virologist, Johan Hultin, travelled to Brevig
Mission, north of the Arctic Circle in Alaska, in the hope
that he would be able to find the virus in the bodies of

victims who had been buried in the permafrost and thereby frozen since 1918. Eighty residents of Brevig had died that year. According to the CDC history, 'Two days in Hultin came across the body of a little girl – her body was still preserved wearing a blue dress, and her hair was adorned with red ribbons.'[107] Hultin and his fellow graduate students obtained lung tissue from her and four others buried at the site, which they transported back to their laboratory in Iowa, but their attempts to grow the virus didn't succeed. Hultin abandoned the quest for 46 years, until one day he read about the efforts of a team led by a molecular pathologist in Washington, DC, Jeffery Taubenberger, to sequence the virus's RNA from a tissue of a serviceman who had died of influenza in 1918 and had been stored at the Armed Forces Institute of Pathology in the city.[108] Taubenberger's team had only managed to reconstruct parts of four of the virus's eight segments. Hultin phoned Taubenberger and proposed returning to Brevig Mission. He paid for the trip with $3,000 of his own savings. Now 72 and equipped with (among other things) his wife's garden shears, he agreed with the village council to try a second excavation. After five days of digging, seven feet into the hard permafrost, he found the perfectly preserved body of an Inuit woman. She was obese and the fat had protected her lungs. Hultin called her 'Lucy'. Shipped to Washington, DC, Lucy's lung tissue contained what the scientists needed. The CDC story shows Hultin standing on top of the gravesite, restored with two crosses that he made at the woodshop of the local school. He is listed as co-author in the first of a series of scientific papers in which the virus's genetic code is identified.[109]

Based on a fuller sequence of the 1918 virus, a team headed by Anne Reid concluded that this virus strain was most closely related to the oldest known swine influenza strain, known as A/sw/Iowa/30. It was later confirmed that the virus had jumped from humans to pigs, not the other way around, and that the virus causing the 2009 'swine flu' pandemic was a descendant.

The next task Reid's team set themselves was reconstructing the virus itself. This was an exercise for a laboratory with all the safeguards needed for biological warfare weapons of mass destruction. Had the virus infected a laboratory worker, or contaminated another influenza strain being researched, or otherwise escaped or been stolen, the implications could have been truly horrendous. This wasn't fanciful – there had been outbreaks of smallpox and other pathogens, including influenza, from laboratories over the years. A team led by Terrence Tumpey at the CDC working under Biosecurity Level 3 was assigned to the task. They worked at night when the laboratories were otherwise deserted. They succeeded in reconstructing the virus – an achievement that Tumpey considered the microbial equivalent of the moon landing.[110] The live virus yielded the complete sequence. It was astonishingly virulent: injected into mice, it replicated at a rate that after four days produced a viral load 39,000 times greater than other influenza strains. But, without comparable data from strains immediately prior to 1918, the origins puzzle was still not solved. Tumpey and his colleagues concluded that the ultimate source of the 1918 virus was an avian virus, but the pathway to the final pandemic form could not be determined: for example, it might have passed through an intermediate mammalian host. Another crucial finding was that there was no single element that made the virus so deadly, but, rather, 'the constellation of all eight genes together make an exceptionally virulent virus.'[111]

It's interesting to note that Tumpey and his colleagues didn't explore more deeply how the 1918 virus could have evolved into such a pathogenic form *within* a human population. They didn't take into account the ecological-evolutionary perspective. In Ewald's critique, 'they still confuse[d] the sources of variation – the mutation and recombination of genes – with the process of evolution by natural selection.'[112]

The next step was constructing a family tree of all influenza strains that have circulated since 1918. Reviewing the evidence in 2009, three of the world's leading infectious disease specialists – David Morens, Jeffery Taubenberger, and Anthony Fauci – concluded:

> [I]t is remarkable not only that direct 'all-eight-gene' descendants of the 1918 virus still circulate in humans as epidemic H1N1 viruses and in swine as epizootic H1N1 viruses, but also that for the last 50 years the original virus and its progeny have continually donated genes to new viruses to cause pandemics, epidemics and epizootics. The novel H1N1 virus associated with the ongoing 2009 pandemic is a fourth-generation descendant of the 1918 virus.[113]

That is a chilling conclusion that compels us to rethink the life history of the disease. In fact the 1918 influenza didn't disappear at all. Instead, the last hundred-plus years of influenza can best be understood as a *single* pandemic. Today, French and Belgian farmers still reap unexploded shells in their fields during every spring ploughing season, and some – a dwindling toll as the decades go by – lose their lives or limbs to this iron harvest. In a similar way, we are falling sick and dying every winter from the viral harvest of that Great War, because the viral progeny of the 1918 pandemic influenza are still with us, reaping their seasonal toll and occasionally recombining to generate a pandemic. Among the legacies of the Flanders trenches is that we are still catching the flu that hatched there.

Track Changes

Concluding her book *Pale Rider*, Laura Spinney suggests it takes a hundred years for the narrative of such a pandemic to distil.[114] It took that long to be able to tell the story from the virus's point of view. So too the story of its human host.

In the writings of the historians, novelists, and poets of Europe and America, influenza was a pandemic outside history and without politics. It was a footnote to the epic convulsion of the Great War and the jarring reconfigurations of the peace that followed. As mentioned, the earliest historian to focus specifically on the pandemic was Alfred Crosby. He was a historian of the political ecology of disease, but he concluded that the impact of the pandemic was found in reams of statistics, and not in public memory.[115] Had he been able to know some of the things that statisticians have since discovered, he might have written (among other things) that the areas of Germany hardest hit by influenza were also those that voted in greatest numbers for the Nazi Party.[116] The sociological equivalent of viral genetic sequencing provides data that confirm the intuitions of those at the time. In 1933, Christopher Isherwood wrote that when the Nazis entered Berlin, 'The whole city lay under an epidemic of discreet, infectious fear. I could feel it, like influenza, in my bones.'[117] Barry commented on that line: '[E]veryone knew what he was talking about.'[118]

Trotsky's locomotive of history was a noisy, clattering steam train – the iron horseman of the apocalypse. The other horsemen were stealthy and quiet. Starvation, the co-equal reaper of death, visited Europe's children and its elderly in the hunger winters of the war. The pale horse and pale rider of influenza moved unnoticed by historians, recognized only three generations after they had passed.

There may be just two public memorials to influenza's dead, but personal memorials are beyond number. The influenza pandemic was many dozens of millions of personal tragedies, a thread woven into the fabric of a hundred million family histories. And so it was not forgotten. In her exploration of the private stories of the pandemic's impact on American lives, Nancy Bristow has shown it was erased from public memory but written into personal and familial memories.[119] Elizabeth Outka spoke to a journalist about researching her book *Viral Modernism*:[120]

Reading letters from survivors of the flu pandemic, one of the things that strikes me over and over again, that's so moving, is that almost every one of them says, 'I never forgot; I never forgot; I never forgot.' [Researching the book], I interviewed one 105-year-old woman who had the flu in Richmond, when she was 8. And in my cheery way, I said something like 'Why do you think people forgot the flu?' And she looked at me like I was crazy. 'We didn't forget! We didn't ignore it! We didn't forget.' She's 105, right? And she was like, 'It never faded – not for us.'[121]

In her book, Outka made the argument that influenza is immanent but unrecognized in modernist literature. For example, T. S. Eliot's *The Waste Land* is suffused with imagery of death, bodies, and rats, and though it mentions neither the war nor the infection, critics have consistently read it through the lens of the war, but never (until her) the pandemic.[122]

Every premature death is a deleted text, a life story untold. Only those who shared the lost hopes and expectations of the person who died will recall the future that was denied. Transfer such human stories to the world stage and the impacts of the pandemic slowly come into focus.

The men who engineered the Russian Revolution were hard of heart and clear in their minds: the great impersonal forces of history shaped class struggle and its outcome. Leon Trotsky was the author of the aphorism that recurs in this and the previous chapter, that war is the locomotive of history – an image that combines industry, motion, and travel along a fixed road of iron. Nonetheless, Vladimir Lenin, asked for a definition of politics, pithily responded, 'who, whom'. For him, a correct understanding of the logic of dialectical materialism needed also an appreciation of the tactics and timing of real politics. In this, the individual counted. Joseph Stalin's infamous words at the time when he was inflicting starvation on Ukraine, that a million deaths are a statistic, was prefaced by saying that one death is a tragedy.

One such death was Yakov Sverdlov, chairman of the All-Russian Central Executive Committee, and thus the *de jure* Soviet head of state, although *de facto* second-in-command to Lenin. Sverdlov contracted influenza in March 1919 and died. He was 33. The loss of this one individual left Lenin – overworked, increasingly unwell, and a theoretician and agitator more than an organizer – bereft of the Revolution's most capable administrator. After some unsatisfactory stop-gaps, Stalin stepped into the vacuum. Trotsky in turn became Stalin's victim. The train of history had switched to a different track, parallel at first but ultimately bending towards a different destination.

Everywhere we look, we find strange deviations, each small but consequential, from the expected path of events, drowned out in the roar of the ending of the war. Mohandas Gandhi was laid low with influenza just as popular anger in India was welling up. Martin Buber was confined to bed just as the Zionist movement demanded decisive action from him. These paths not taken have a pattern in common: those who expected to command decisions found themselves instead following events, rushing to catch up and never quite making it. Perhaps the most consequential lurch on history's track was President Woodrow Wilson's incapacitation in Paris at a critical juncture in the peace talks.[123] Professional historians have hesitated to conclude that it was influenza,[124] but the evidence is compelling, if circumstantial. The White House butler, Irwin 'Ike' Hoover, provides a first-hand account of Wilson's illness, and that 'something queer was happening in his mind'.[125] It is likely that influenza so debilitated the physical and mental capacity of the American president that he abandoned his principle of 'peace without victory' in favour of the retributive approach towards Germany that France was pushing. Hoover concludes, 'One thing was certain; he was never the same after this little spell of illness.'[126] The consequences of his capitulation were foreseen at the time by his appalled advisers. As Isherwood felt in Berlin 14 years later, along with the Nazis also came the chill of influenza.

Twentieth-century urban civilization dodged a viral bullet. In the previous century, the logic of recurrent cholera had dictated that cities be constructed – and often rebuilt from their foundations – as sanitation systems. For some years, driven by miasmatism and fear of tuberculosis, fresh-air movements had urged building design that maximized air circulation. A history of central heating notes how fear of influenza fanned the fresh air fervour: 'You can see it in the engineering books published after 1920. The authors wrote of the Fresh Air Movement and cautioned engineers to specify boilers and radiators that will be large enough to heat the building on the coldest day of the year, with the windows open.'[127] However, because the 1918 influenza was a hit-and-run pandemic, so too the reorganization of public space was ephemeral. Metro systems, theatres, offices, hotels, and apartment blocks continued to be built with only minor adjustments, and a few decades later, forgetful architects designed systems for heating and ventilation based entirely on recycled air and windows that can't be opened. Instead, when governments began thinking about influenza pandemic preparedness, they did so on a model of identifying and eliminating the microbial enemy *before* it could breach our defences. No-one wanted to think about what a pandemic respiratory pathogen might do if it took up permanent residence in the conducive ecology of our cities.

The Great Influenza is the paradigmatic pandemic, against which we measure all pathogenic threats, actual and anticipated. But it is too big to fit into any storyline. The scale of the 1918 influenza is microscopic and global, momentary and age-long – and personal. This it shares with the Black Death of the 14th century, which left a legacy of disbelief, which historians could only begin to sift after half a millennium had passed. In her history of that calamitous century, Barbara Tuchman notes the 'vacuum of comment' about the plague in the political chronicles of the time.[128] Norman Cantor concludes *In the Wake of the Plague* with reflections on the significance of the late-medieval *danse macabre* and the 'new era of death consciousness, funeral ritualization, extravagant guilt and macabre imagining' which 'facilitated the incapacity for human responses to the Black Death'.[129] Phillip Ziegler ended his seminal history of the medieval Great Plague with these words: 'The generation that survived the plague could not believe but did not dare deny.'[130] Ziegler depicts the late-medieval individual as a figure 'as if silhouetted against a background of Wagnerian tempest'. But this was not a hero defying the storm. 'Rather, it was as if he wandered in from another play [*King Lear*]: an Edgar crying plaintively, "Poor Tom's a-cold; poor Tom's a-cold!" and seeking what shelter he could against the elements.' Ziegler concludes, 'Poor Tom survived, but he was never to be quite the same again.'[131]

4

Who, Whom: HIV/AIDS

The Ugandan singer Philly Bongole Lutaaya wrote his greatest song when he was dying of AIDS, about dying of AIDS. He called it 'Alone and Frightened'. He performed it live just once, in October 1989 at a concert in Kampala's Nakivubo Stadium. Lutaaya walked unsteadily to the stage but his voice was strong. He started solo, lamenting his isolation and lack of love and sex. Singing this song gave a public face to AIDS in Uganda. People talked about him and this new and bewildering virus on buses and in bars, market-places, and churches.[1]

'Alone and Frightened' isn't usually listed among the compilations of top AIDS songs, which include laments, elegies, and ballads (Leonard Cohen's 'Everybody Knows', Elton John's 'The Last Song', and Bruce Springsteen's 'Streets of Philadelphia'). Lutaaya's song is not like any of those. It becomes a duet. A woman singer – her name isn't given anywhere in the recordings – responds, reaching out with a voice of love. When the chorus joins, it becomes an anthem, summoning the audience to sing too. Among European and American singers, the only comparable track is Annie Lennox's 'Sing', which she released 18 years later as a goodwill ambassador for UNAIDS (the United Nations special agency for coordinating the international response to HIV and AIDS). It is a song of joy and hope that Lennox performs jointly with African singers and dancers, and it includes lyrics in South African languages. In short, it sounds African – like Lutaaya's song.

'Alone and Fighting' is also a fighting song, in which Lutaaya calls for everyone to stand up and fight against AIDS. If this is the language of war, it's about a very different kind of war to Europe's wars of mass conscripts and territorial conquest. Lutaaya's previous hit song, 'Born in Africa', was a celebration of Africa and African freedom. As a proud pan-Africanist, when he called for a 'fight' against AIDS, he would have been thinking of a people's war of liberation, in the tradition of Che Guevara's words, 'At the risk of seeming ridiculous, let me say that the true revolutionary is guided by a great feeling of love.'

In reality, guerrilla wars of this kind are nasty, brutal, and long. In Uganda, the recent war of resistance had been against a post-colonial dictator. Lutaaya sang 'Alone and Frightened' shortly after guerrilla fighters led by a charismatic young revolutionary named Yoweri Museveni had won power and their vision of a new Uganda was shining brightly. It soon began to fade. Like other liberators in power, Museveni liked power more than democracy. Lutaaya didn't live long enough to see that. The Nakivubo concert was his last. He died in a Kampala hospital on 15 December 1989. He was 38.

Disease and war look different when seen from outside the citadels of privilege and expertise. Cholera was a pandemic of colonial conquest that the colonists finally succeeded in confining to the colonies. Africans and Asians were quick to see pandemic influenza as a sickness of empire and war, and correctly so. Pandemic HIV and AIDS are also best understood if we begin in Africa. Like every other pandemic, it was unexpected in its own way. People suffering from advanced AIDS are emaciated and Ugandans called the disease 'slim'.

Repurposing English words or phrases to mock dark current events is a speciality of Ugandan humour. 'Slim' is the only known vernacular term for AIDS before American clinicians named the syndrome in 1982. A year earlier, in their first reports of the mysterious disease, doctors had called it 'gay-related immune deficiency syndrome', which was an inauspicious (and false) conflating of a sexual identity with a disease. The Euro-American medical establishment might have done better with a sense of irony borrowed from a former colony. The emergence of a new infectious pathogen came as a surprise to medical science – though in retrospect, what was more surprising was the complacency of the public health establishment.

HIV travelled around the world because enough people were connected in ways that made it possible for a virus to spread silently through needles and through sex, and because the microbe was helped on its way by a string of accidents of history. HIV is classed as a 'lentivirus' – one that acts slowly – and the pandemic is, overall, very slow moving, though there are occasional bursts of local acceleration. Influenza's spread is mapped in weeks; HIV's in years. It took about 25 years for the worldwide curve of infections to be flattened and we're now on a downslope, though there is nothing automatic about a continuing decline. One medical demographer estimated the pandemic as an '130-year event', which may turn out to be optimistic.[2] Once again, the textbook terminologies don't fit well. In its everyday usage, an 'epidemic' refers to a fast-moving event, in contrast to an ever-present 'endemic' disease, so perhaps we should re-label HIV a 'novel endemic'.

With the insights provided by genomic sequencing of HIV and its ancestors in other apes, we now know that the strain of HIV that was causing 'slim' in Uganda was transmitted from a chimpanzee in south-east Cameroon to a human being in or before 1920, and by the 1930s it was circulating in the twin towns of Brazzaville and Léopoldville (now Kinshasa) opposite one another on the banks of the

Congo river. It wasn't named at the time, but it wasn't invisible either. Jacques Pepin, who has picked through the archives of colonial medicine in search of clues for the origins of AIDS, has found descriptions of cases suggestive of AIDS among the men forced to labour on the Congo–Océan railway in 1931.[3] Pathologists described a syndrome, an unknown tropical disease afflicting Africans. It provoked their professional curiosity but not much more. Work conditions on the railway were scandalously bad, described by one contemporary report in these words: 'Spent, mistreated . . . , injured, emaciated, desolate, the blacks die en masse.'[4] In a similar way, AIDS in central Africa half a century later might also have gone unremarked by the medical establishment, at least for some years, were it not for the sudden and baffling emergence of the syndrome among gay men in North American cities.

Since AIDS was recognized in 1981, it has infected about 75 million people around the world and killed just under half of them. It is best seen not as a single event, but as a set of overlapping outbreaks affecting different populations: gay men in the United States and Europe; haemophiliacs; injecting drug users; sex workers and their clients; and in southern and eastern Africa, a 'hyper-endemic' among the heterosexual population, with a fifth or more of the entire adult population infected with the virus at any one time.

As with other pandemics, where the data and evidence were missing, political narratives wrote the lines that joined the dots. In the case of HIV and AIDS, people affected by the pandemic contested the authoritative version and wrote different new storylines that included liberation, equity, and democracy.

Cohabiting with HIV

The human immunodeficiency virus (HIV) follows a different kind of adaptive strategy to our two previous microbial protagonists. It's stealthy. Almost like a shadow, HIV is a quiet intruder that steals into its host's home. For the host there's little disturbance at first as the virus finds its place – viral levels surge a few weeks after initial infection. The human host hardly notices those mild symptoms. For the virus, however, this is anything but incidental. In fact, it's HIV's main chance to slip into new homes. HIV is a self-effacing pathogen: that early sickness mustn't be severe enough to stop the host having sex, and after that it lurks unnoticed for as long as 10 years, its job already done. The host continues his or her life without paying any attention, and HIV returns the favour.

To follow HIV, we need to follow the question of who does what with whom. The virus travels with blood and sex direct from one person to another. They may be sharing intimacy and pleasure. One person may be exercising power over another, or it may be a commercial transaction. Or HIV can take a free ride on a medical procedure.

Transmission by injection is by far the most efficient mode of transmitting HIV – it has an entry pass straight into the bloodstream and even a very small dose is enough to infect someone new. Transmission through open cuts and abrasions was important for cross-species infections and is an occasional risk among humans. Sex is the commonest form of transmission. Some forms of sex are more advantageous to HIV than others: anal sex is more risky than vaginal sex, and HIV travels more readily if either partner has a different sexually transmitted infection such as gonorrhoea. Uncircumcised men are slightly better for the virus than circumcised. HIV is also transmitted from mothers to children, *in utero* or through breastfeeding. That's a special terrible human tragedy, but for the virus it's a dead end because HIV-positive children don't often transmit the virus to others. In what follows, I focus on HIV in adults.

Once HIV has found its way in, it can't be dislodged. Then, after something between five and fifteen years, it makes its presence felt in a sly manner. Like a night-time poltergeist, it opens the door to sundry pathogenic passers-by roaming the neighbourhood, which are the ones that actually disturb the house and ultimately wreck it. This means that cohabiting with HIV is ultimately fatal. As those other pathogens crowd in, HIV itself multiplies again. Although people with AIDS-related diseases are very infectious, they're less likely to be sexually active, so for the virus this second round of transmission chances is really only a last-chance party.

In Africa, the most common of these opportunistic infections is tuberculosis – a particular danger because it is a widespread dormant infection that usually awakens when its host's immune system is weak. Africa's AIDS epidemic has brought with it a huge resurgence of TB, and (of particular concern) the emergence of multi-drug-resistant strains of TB.

HIV is a transactional pathogen. For it to survive in a human population, it needs a lot of people to share bodily fluids. Ideal is a group of injecting drug users passing around a single needle, or a clinic reusing unsterilized equipment. But even some initially favourable ecologies for HIV may result mostly in dead-end infections. For example, people infected in a rural clinic may infect their partners and children but HIV is likely to remain within that circle. The infected people need to have intimate transactions with others in their most infectious period a few weeks after contracting the virus, and those others with others. If a drug user is also selling sex, for example, then his or her clients may well become infected and pass HIV to their spouses, partners, or other sex workers. If we're dealing with sexual transmission, what's crucial is that there should be a *web* of sexual transactions. A *string* of partnerships won't do: an HIV-positive person who has six relationships, each lasting years, may transmit the virus, but it will spread much more slowly. A web of contacts is a different matter.[5] Gay men in European and North American cities who hung out in clubs and bathhouses around 1980 formed such a web.

Most attention has been given to unprotected anal sex as a transmission route; just as important was frequent partner change.

It's the same for heterosexual sex. An HIV-positive man who visits a sex worker every week, rotating among his favourites in three or four towns, who in turn have a dozen clients whom they regularly have sex with, is a node in a web through which the virus will spread. The crucial 'sustaining population' that harbours the virus over time isn't actually the sex workers, but the men who control the sex trade, such as pimps, policemen, and gangsters who provide 'protection', and the most privileged clients.[6] This is a common pattern around the world. A young woman who has a 'sugar daddy' who helps pay her college fees, as well as a boyfriend, each of them having another regular sexual partner, is a member of another high-risk web. If the man is 20 years older than his girlfriend, that means that the virus is shared with a younger generation. Unfortunately for the people of eastern and southern Africa, this combination of gendered power that exploits young women, open-ended sexual networks, and geographical mobility is common there.[7]

Many pathogens evolve towards lower virulence: it's usually better for a parasite for its host to stay alive. HIV is prone to mutation, and exhibits 'the highest recorded biological mutation rate currently known to science'.[8] However, it has characteristics that minimize the constraints that would otherwise reduce its virulence.[9] In particular, most transmission occurs long before any AIDS-related symptoms develop. For HIV, the symptoms of AIDS are secondary.

HIV's Thread

For a pathogen to go pandemic, the thread of its biography must pass through the eyes of several needles. Pandemic HIV did this four times: a virulent strain made the zoonotic jump, and shortly afterwards it became endemic in a human community. The thread then divided into two, each of which generated a distinct but simultaneous epidemic.

The pandemic strain is HIV-1 (group M). There is also HIV-2, which is much less virulent, and many of those infected live out their lives without even knowing they have it. There are three other strains of HIV-1, known as 'N', 'O', and 'P', which are rare. These other members of the family are interesting to virologists because they help in constructing HIV's genealogy and understanding why HIV-1(M) became endemic in west-central Africa and then pandemic. And once it became established in humans, this strain also evolved a score or so of subtypes, by mutation (HIV doesn't proofread its copies) and recombination (two subtypes sharing their genes when they meet in a single host).

The ancestor of HIV is simian immunodeficiency virus (SIV), which has a natural reservoir in monkeys in west-central Africa.[10] Almost for sure, SIV jumped to human beings many times in the past, presumably through the open wound on a hunter's hand or forearm as he killed or butchered a monkey. That hunter might have then infected his partner, and she might have passed the virus on to her child. Perhaps a few others were infected too. In a small, isolated forest community, the outbreak would have ended there. Also, most strains of SIV weren't virulent enough to become epidemic in a local population.

There are 13 known instances of SIV zoonosis that have germinated HIV lineages among human beings.[11] Nine HIV strains leapt directly from sooty mangabey monkeys, which live in the forests of the west African coast, stretching from Senegal to Côte d'Ivoire. Their SIV is identical to HIV-2, so named because it was isolated in 1985 in Senegal, soon after the identification of HIV, which was then reclassified as 'HIV-1'. Perhaps half of those people infected with HIV-2 live out their natural lifespan as it has a very long latency period and low lethality. Four HIV strains moved through other primates as intermediary hosts before humans. These are identified as HIV-1, originating in monkeys in the central

African rainforests of Cameroon, Gabon, and Congo. The SIV in these monkey populations has also infected chimpanzees and gorillas in the past, presumably because larger primates hunt monkeys for food, and they suffer bites and scratches when killing their prey which are sites of infection. Chimpanzees also fall sick and die from simian AIDS, and it's one reason (alongside hunting and loss of habitat) that populations of chimpanzees in the wild are dwindling and endangered.[12] Today's four strains of HIV-1 in humans arose from separate zoonotic events, two from chimpanzees and two from gorillas.[13] Three of these are localized and less virulent. One is the pandemic HIV-1 (group M). This appears to be a recombinant version of two SIV strains that emerged in a chimpanzee, several thousand years ago.[14] In the early 20th century, a human being, probably a hunter, became infected. This was HIV's first threading of the needle.

In the first 25 years of pandemic HIV/AIDS, the species jump from other apes to humans was accepted as another microbial 'just so' story – something new and pathogenic out of Africa that needed no further explanation. The exoticism and distastefulness of chimpanzee–human transmission was a reason to leave this topic alone: AIDS specialists were already dealing with big enough problems of stigma and discrimination that an origins story involving eating our closest primate relatives was a path into the rainforest best left undisturbed.[15]

This left a second question unexplored: how did a local zoonosis become an outbreak that turned pandemic? We know that HIV is hard to transmit: could just one 'patient zero' have infected enough people? In the opening pages of his account of the North American epidemic among gay men, Randy Shilts introduced the Canadian flight attendant Gaétan Dugas as the index case for HIV.[16] Shilts didn't intend to promote Dugas from an exemplar of the epidemic into the individual culprit: rather, this was the angle that the book's promoters and reviewers picked up on because it was a more dramatic story.[17] Where it was correct was that quite exceptional levels of sexual activity with a high risk of transmitting HIV were needed to seed an epidemic, and Dugas, who had hundreds of such encounters each year and was also highly mobile, showed how this was possible. But it actually didn't happen that way: sequencing HIV's genome and reconstructing the timeline of its evolution using its molecular clock, we now know that HIV first came to North America in approximately 1969.[18] And of course, even if Dugas had been the gay community's first superspreader, it didn't explain why the virus had *already* spread in central Africa.

In a 1992 article in *Rolling Stone*, Tom Curtis proposed a controversial theory of HIV origins.[19] He argued that in the 1950s, medical scientists involved in polio vaccination campaigns running a laboratory near Stanleyville (now Kisangani) in Congo had used a culture from primate kidneys to cultivate oral polio vaccines and had unwittingly used SIV-infected monkeys and thereby spread HIV. The medical establishment lined up to dismiss the hypothesis as frivolous, dangerous, and irrelevant. The doctor in charge of the facility sued *Rolling Stone* and won a retraction and apology. The magazine ran up hundreds of thousands of dollars in lawyers' costs, and it took a brave writer to revisit the polio vaccine argument. The journalist Ed Hooper did so in his 1999 book *The River*.[20] We now know that Curtis and Hooper were wrong: the SIV ancestor of HIV originated much further west and jumped to humans much earlier, so that polio vaccines were not the culprit.[21] But there was something disturbing about the haste with which the medical establishment tried to dismiss Curtis and Hooper as amateurs peddling conspiracies.[22] The amateurs were onto something.

Transmission by needle into the bloodstream is a far more efficient way of spreading HIV than sexual practices of any kind. There is strong circumstantial evidence that this happened with HIV-2 in west Africa. Recall that HIV-2 is much less virulent and remains symptomless in about half of those infected. This means that people who acquired HIV-2 in the 1950s and 1960s, at the time of mass campaigns of inoculation in those countries, were still alive when testing for HIV became widespread 30 years later. Among the epidemiological curiosities of HIV-2 is that in 2000 infection rates among elderly west Africans were far higher than among younger people, the opposite of what one would expect in a generalized epidemic of sexually transmitted infection. One possible explanation for the anomaly is that HIV-2 spread widely in Guinea-Bissau during the liberation war in the 1960s and early 1970s due to soldiers and guerillas having sex with lots of different women.[23] What we know about HIV transmission patterns during war makes this very unlikely (see below). Much more credible is that the virus was spread through unsterilized injections.[24] We know that there were epidemics of hepatitis spread by contaminated injections, and outbreaks of HIV-1 in Romania, Libya, and China caused by poorly sterilized needles and syringes or contaminated blood supplies. Careful examination of evidence from contemporary Africa also implicates exposure during health care in a frighteningly high proportion of cases.[25]

The most exhaustive investigation into the origins of pandemic HIV has been undertaken by Jacques Pepin.[26] He combines the information from reconstructions of HIV's genome, SIV genomes, the retrieval of blood and tissue samples from the earliest AIDS cases, the historical sociology of public health, and epidemiological modelling. Pepin argues that the sexual transmission hypothesis on its own cannot account for the pattern of spread: the numbers simply don't add up. Instead, iatrogenic transmission through colonial medical practices was the factor that inadvertently amplified a localized HIV-1 outbreak into enduring endemic status in the twin cities of Brazzaville and Léopoldville. In the interwar period, officials at the Pasteur Institutes in Brazzaville and Dakar (known as 'Pastorians') organized huge campaigns targeted at specific diseases. Today we would call these 'vertical' programmes to distinguish them from 'horizontal' support to an all-purpose health infrastructure. According to the historian Aro Velmet, the imperial authorities liked them because they were low cost and standardized and gave a plausible imitation of a *mission civilisatrice* without having to provide the entitlement to state services expected by citizens of the metropolis.[27] The first such campaign, which became the model, was aimed at controlling Trypanosomiasis (sleeping sickness). This disease is transmitted by tsetse flies and was common across Africa's forest zones. Endemic Trypanosomiasis risked making some districts uninhabitable, thereby depriving the colonialists of their labour force. It also threatened European settlers. Over 15 years (1920–35), a region-wide campaign to suppress sleeping sickness was led by the hyperactive Dr Eugène Jamot, whose methods earned the special moniker *La Jamotique*.[28] These were a dramatic performance of medical colonial power and were popularized in France, as described by Velmet:

Films such as *Sleeping Sickness* (Alfred Chaumel, 1930) conventionally began with a series of maps, laying out the scope of the empire and its terrains ('endemic,' 'epidemic,' and 'endoepidemic') where the battle against diseases was to be fought. Chaumel represented the mass treatment efforts of the Pastorian Eugène Jamot as military campaigns: he juxtaposed shots of nurses, auxiliaries, and doctors waiting in formation for patients with images of tribesmen emerging from the brush in the hundreds to present themselves for treatment, resembling a military parade or inspection. The camera lingered long on Jamot himself, following the bacteriologist as he oversaw the various procedures, corrected the technique of auxiliaries, and made sure statistics were properly recorded. Jamot appeared as a general overseeing the military inspection, an impression further reinforced by shots of the French tricolor at the end of the film.[29]

La Jamotique achieved its goal and its commander was honoured as the man who conquered sleeping sickness. Later campaigns against syphilis and yellow fever followed the same model. All utilized mass injection, reusing equipment without sterilization. So too did the medical inspections for army recruits when the Free French mobilized in central Africa in 1940. In fact this was routine colonial medical practice. Pepin quotes Dr Paul Beheyt, a doctor working in Congo in the 1950s, who wrote that:

> The Congo contains various health institutions (maternity centres, hospitals, dispensaries, etc.) where every day local nurses give dozens, even hundreds, of injections in conditions such that sterilisation of the needle or the syringe is impossible. ... Used syringes are simply rinsed, first with water, then with alcohol or ether, and are ready for a new patient. The syringe is used from one patient to the next, occasionally retaining small quantities of infectious blood.[30]

Jamot and his successors inadvertently created an artificial ecology ideally conducive for the iatrogenic amplification of HIV. It would have taken just a few cases of contamination to spread the virus to new populations where it could become endemic. Unlike the investigations by Curtis and Hooper, Pepin's analysis has been taken seriously.[31] But the public health establishment doesn't want to face its discomforting message: that it might share responsibility for HIV/AIDS.

The second accelerant of HIV was the colonial reorganization of sex. Europeans in Africa created dual economies: capitalist enclaves and rural reserves. Where the colonizers set up plantations, mines, work camps, ports, and administrative centres, they needed African labourers. But they didn't want to pay wages sufficient to support a family, and they didn't want to have to administer a complete community either, whose leaders might demand welfare and civil rights. Instead they set up native quarters where male workers could stay for as long as their labour was needed, after which they would be sent 'home' to villages. This extreme social engineering wasn't viable, even where the profits were highest and the administration fiercest, such as South Africa's mine workers' hostels. At minimum, the all-male labour force needed at least a faint imitation of the comforts of home: food, laundry, companionship, and sex.[32] Women slipped inside these enclaves or lived on their fringes. They were often called 'prostitutes' and sometimes 'free women'. Many solely sold sex; some managed bars and tea houses; others had more stable relationships with higher-status men. These societies, or fragments of societies, aren't either 'traditional' or 'modern'; they are neither 'urban' nor 'rural' – they are a special creation. The sexual networks within them are implicitly transactional, temporary, and confined to the artificial circumstances of the enclave.

This is where HIV became endemic between the 1920s and the 1950s: in the railway work camps (where those earliest cases of AIDS-like syndromes were observed) and in the colonial capitals on the banks of the Congo river. At that early stage, HIV didn't follow the explosive pattern that was seen in cities such Nairobi in the 1980s, when it accelerated from a tiny number of infections to an epidemic affecting one in five of the population. It was probably more like the pattern of low-level endemicity seen in contemporary west African cities, where infections are concentrated among sex workers and their clients.[33]

The two accelerants – iatrogenic transmission and sexual networks – intersected. It's very likely that clinics for treating venereal diseases spread HIV. In the 1920s, missionaries and colonial administrators became worried over what they believed was epidemic syphilis in central Africa – a medical emergency mixed with a moral panic.[34] They started big campaigns to prevent people who had suspected latent syphilis from developing the symptomatic disease. Most people who got positive results on syphilis tests actually had antibodies from childhood yaws (a disfiguring bacterial skin infection commonly acquired by children playing together or eating with unwashed fingers from a shared plate) or the similar symptoms of a disease known as bejel (a form of syphilis transmitted by non-sexual contact, for example by sharing domestic utensils).[35] Regardless, all were injected with anti-syphilitic drugs on the grounds that it was better to err on the side of caution. There's a sick irony that the missionary-imperial dread of African sexuality, made potentially pathogenic through colonially constructed male labour enclaves, was made actually pathogenic through policies intended to suppress venereal disease.

This is the second needle threaded by HIV: how it became endemic in colonial cities. Intriguingly, given HIV's later accelerated spread elsewhere in Africa, its levels remained low in Congo for decades and have remained so until today. It peaked at about 5 per cent of the adult population between 2000 and 2005 – very high by the standards of anywhere except sub-Saharan Africa, but curiously suppressed compared to neighbouring countries. Despite the collapse of the health system since the outbreak of the first Congo war in 1996, alongside enormous social disruption including well-documented sexual violence, the rate of HIV has declined steadily to its current level of about 1 per cent.

From the reconstruction of the genetics of HIV, we know that the virus spread within Congo along two main arteries: eastwards up the river to Kisangani and south-east by road and rail to the mining centres of Mbuyi-Maji and Kisangani.[36] It was endemic in these towns by the 1950s, though still unrecognized in medical reporting. HIV-1, group M, subtype A continued travelling east, reaching Rwanda and Uganda in the 1960s.[37] HIV-1, group M, subtype C evolved in the mining centres. It didn't penetrate the broader Congolese population, but it spread throughout southern Africa, accelerating in the 1980s.[38] Today, subtype C is the dominant one in southern Africa, responsible for about half of the world's total HIV infections. How it spread explosively – suddenly reaching 20 or 30 per cent of all adults in eastern and southern Africa – is the third needle threaded.

At this time, the biography of HIV divides, with a separate thread crossing the Atlantic. Over the years, a few individual non-Africans had been infected with HIV and there was a smattering of cases of aid workers, sailors, and others who presented with AIDS-like symptoms in European hospitals years before AIDS was recognized. Newly independent Congo also hosted several thousand Haitian professionals, brought in because the country needed a civil service and the Belgians had neglected to train any Congolese. Haitians spoke French and had pan-African sensibilities harking back to their own revolution. One of these Haitian *coopérants* acquired a rare subtype (HIV-1, group M, subtype B) which he took back to Haiti in about 1966. The virological genetic evidence points to a single founder event: just one person, presumably a man, was patient zero for the Americas.[39] Conceding that the trail of microbial evidence becomes thinner after this point, Pepin argues that it is likely that the crucial accelerant in Haiti – and also the factor that introduced HIV to the United States – was a medical blood supply company called Hemo-Caribbean run by a crony of François 'Papa Doc' Duvalier.[40] Without such a powerful multiplier, he argues, HIV in Haiti would almost certainly have died out.

Hemo-Caribbean, or something with a similar formula of amplification, is the fourth needle threaded by HIV. Subtype B went on to cause epidemics in America, Europe, Australasia, and elsewhere among homosexual men, injecting drug users, sex workers and their clients, and wherever unscrupulous or careless medical authorities failed to take precautions to ensure that blood supplies were screened and protected. For gay men, injecting drug users, and sex workers, AIDS was an existential threat: to their individual lives and to them as communities. Each of these epidemics deserves its own special analysis, but because they are so varied and generalization is so difficult, in my account here I will treat them only in passing. Instead I will focus on southern and eastern Africa.

This is the story up to 1981, the reconstruction of the history of a virus before it was recognized by medicine. It wasn't until 30 years later, and the development of viral genomic sequencing and sophisticated epidemiological modelling, that it became possible to tell it. The biggest lesson of that story is that nothing was inevitable about AIDS. To the contrary, the odds against the virus were very long indeed and a string of extraordinary circumstances was needed to make HIV viable in human populations.

After Austerity, after Conflict, after Apartheid

The HIV/AIDS epidemics exploded across eastern and southern Africa in the 1990s just as those countries were emerging from a long and ravaging economic recession. South Africans were shedding the shackles of Apartheid. The African National Congress (ANC) had been unbanned and was on its way to the historic election of Nelson Mandela as president in 1994. Their immediate neighbours were celebrating the end of the devastating proxy wars between the racist government in South Africa and the majority-ruled 'frontline states' – conflicts that had blighted the southern third of the continent for a generation. Almost everywhere, the media was becoming free and multi-party politics was displacing stagnant authoritarianism. It was known as Africa's 'democracy wave'. The future was bright, but the future was also AIDS.

Uganda was the first country to suffer an explosive AIDS epidemic, and unlike Congo, it became horribly visible. Its epicentre was in the south-west of the country, where HIV multiplied in the 1970s and 1980s in a thickly settled rural area where people's livelihoods came from farming, fishing, and an informal economy known as *magendo*, including smuggling and a host of illegal and semi-legal activities that eked an income at the margins.[41] When HIV testing became available, the seroprevalence rates were shocking: 25 per cent and rising in the worst-hit communities. Uganda's national HIV levels hit 10 per cent in 1990.

This was a time of economic crisis and political turmoil, including the dictatorship of Idi Amin (in power 1971–9), a border war between Uganda and Tanzania followed by a Tanzanian invasion (1978–9), and a series of civil wars that culminated in the victory of the guerrilla army headed by Yoweri Museveni in 1986. When Museveni took power, Uganda was in ruins, the first African country (along with Chad) to be described as a 'failed state'. AIDS was written into this script. Journalists' reporting from the country chimed with 'heart of darkness' clichés:

> The heart of Africa is stricken. The 'AIDS belt' is spreading, and the disease that has already claimed the lives of thousands of men, women, and children will claim millions more. *Vanity Fair* sent Alex Shoumatoff on a journey of exploration along the equator, where he met the fatalistic bar girls of Kinshasa, the exhausted doctors of war-shattered Uganda, the folk healers of Guinea-Bissau, and the plague-ridden smugglers of Lake Victoria. Is this a nightmare vision of our own future?[42]

Shoumatoff himself played up the theme, imagining himself as a Victorian explorer: 'How curious it would be, I think, if the source of the Nile and the source of AIDS prove to be one and the same, that huge teeming lake deep in the dangerous heart of darkest Africa.' A few years later, when the Cold War was over but Africa was facing new crises of state collapse, the journalist Robert Kaplan updated the trope. His article was entitled 'The Coming Anarchy: How scarcity, crime, overpopulation, tribalism, and disease are rapidly destroying the social fabric of our planet'.[43]

Ignore for now the histrionics and stereotyping. AIDS had already become an emblem and symptom of every kind of disorder, a disease of war, chaos, and transgression. At first sight, it seems obvious that war and HIV ought to march together. Armies and sexually transmitted infections have long been intimate fellow-travellers. Anecdotes about very high rates of HIV among soldiers – two to five times as high as among civilians – were taken as evidence for military epidemics. There is evidence that the virus moved with Tanzanian soldiers when they invaded Uganda. Among the founders of Museveni's guerrilla army, more died from AIDS than in combat.[44] But the links between conflict and AIDS become less clear the closer we look,[45] and as better comparative data have become available, researchers have concluded that civil war actually *lowers* HIV prevalence, albeit modestly. The reasons for this include the recruitment pool for infantry armies (young men from villages, a demographic category with low HIV prevalence); the prompt adoption by armies of compulsory testing for HIV and stern disciplinary measures against those found positive (contrary to best human rights practice, but effective nonetheless); and the ways in which the disruptions to trade, movement, and residence patterns during war don't tend to create the kinds of interlinked sexual networks that facilitate HIV transmission.[46] Rape definitely increases the risk of HIV transmission, both for the individual victim and, in cases of mass rape, for the population.[47] In some appalling cases, such as Rwanda, rapists deliberately set out to infect their victims.[48] These episodes register among the most appalling atrocities, but their epidemiological significance is less, both because they are rare and because survivors of atrocity rape are usually not sexually active in their infectious stage. As mentioned, despite Congo ranking at the top of every war-related indicator, it hasn't suffered a high-level generalized HIV epidemic. In the Ugandan case, we simply can't tell whether the war and social crisis of the 1970s and 1980s accelerated HIV, hindered it, or had no overall effect. What we can say is that the AIDS-and-anarchy storyline misled journalists, public health experts, and politicians.

Uganda's epidemic was also unusual in that its epicentre was a rural area. Comparable HIV epidemics struck villages on the Tanzanian and Kenyan shores of Lake Victoria and in a few other places such as the home villages of migrant workers, all of which turned out to be exceptions to the usual pattern of HIV concentrations in cities, along main roads, and in populations of managed labour. But the fact that the first acknowledged African epidemic occurred in villages fed the scare that hyper-endemic HIV was a risk for *any* community, and that HIV levels of 25 per cent or even more represented the natural trajectory of the epidemic. In retrospect, that wasn't warranted: HIV needed special conditions to reach those levels.

Those special conditions existed in near-perfect combination (for the virus) where there was a legacy of the colonial-era labour enclaves. Where that system had been enforced on the largest possible scale – South Africa and its immediate neighbours – the epidemic moved fastest and reached the highest levels. The whole southern African region resembled a set of circuits waiting for the electricity to be turned on, and the switch was thrown when people began to move more in the 1980s and 1990s. There were plenty of wrinkles and anomalies – Uganda was one – but the overall pattern is consistent over time and space, and also consistent with the earlier history of HIV in Congo. The motor was that enough people had unprotected sex with more than one partner, and those partnerships were concurrent, creating a web. It took some time before this straightforward epidemiological fact was acknowledged. This delay mattered a great deal because in the meantime a lot of AIDS messages, policies, and programmes were based on the wrong premises.[49]

Among some specific groups, such as sex workers and injecting drug users, HIV can increase at an exponential rate, going from a handful of cases to a third or more of the population in a year or less. In southern Africa, this exponential increase rolled through an entire population. It could be represented as a wave on a graph – or, to be more precise, as two waves. First came an invisible wave of infections. This was followed with a relentless inevitability by the terribly visible wave of sickness and death. Those who could read the graph knew that the second wave was coming and nothing could be done to stop it. Like a seismologist standing on a beach emptied of its water, knowing that a tsunami is coming and that it's not possible to run fast or far enough to get to high ground, the South African economist Alan Whiteside used the double curve to tell the story of what lay in store if HIV transmission were not controlled.[50]

This was terrifying for southern Africans, and many theories were propounded, including various 'wrath of God' explanations and the 'Operation INFEKTION' story put about by Soviet and East German intelligence that the virus had been engineered by the CIA. Four other accounts deserve our attention because they were much more influential.

The first was a rerun of the colonial moral panic about African sexuality: the argument that Africans have more sex, and types of sex that are riskier for HIV. Sexual practices differ across cultures, so this kind of explanation shouldn't be dismissed out of hand as racist, though culturalist explanations for disease are often made by racists.[51] African leaders had their own variant on this panic, appropriating the colonial-missionary script that defined homosexuality as 'non-African' and preaching conservative sexual mores.[52] More important is to ask why certain kinds of webs of sexual interaction existed in the first place, and by far the most cogent explanation for this lies in the historical demography of colonial labour practices.

A second explanation is that AIDS is a disease of poverty. What's right about this is that if the African countries where the first AIDS cases occurred had been rich nations, the disease would have been investigated, named, and responded to much more quickly. Even if those countries had retained the health care infrastructure that they had built up in the 1960s and 1970s, before economic crisis and austerity measures, they would have been better placed. These truths were pressed into service to make the point that African countries needed more aid money, especially for health, and that the 'structural adjustment' policies imposed by the World Bank,

International Monetary Fund, and western creditors were a cruel error. There's a lot to be said for each of these arguments, but they don't add up to an explanation for why HIV exploded where it did, and why it didn't explode where it didn't. Countries like Chad, Sierra Leone, and Somalia, for example, were in the path of HIV, and were poorer and with worse health care, but only suffered epidemics concentrated among sex workers and their clients. Tellingly, none of them had the combination of colonial-style labour management and an economic rebound.

Explanation three is that the epidemic was driven by war. As explained above, this isn't true in general. However, the *end* of southern Africa's wars with the ending of Apartheid was conducive to the transmission of HIV. The return of refugees and the opening up of commercial routes into areas formerly cut off by war are opportunities for the virus.[53] The Apartheid government used irregular proxies stationed in the Caprivi Strip in northern Namibia to fight its 'dirty wars' in Angola and Namibia and to destabilize other countries, and when those soldiers returned to South Africa they carried HIV with them.[54] ANC fighters also contracted HIV at their bases in Tanzania and Angola and brought the virus home. What Horace Campbell has called the 'patriarchal model of liberation'[55] was rhetorically committed to women's equality and allowed female members of the vanguard to take senior positions, but it subjugated women. I remember that when a delegation from the South-West African People's Organization (SWAPO) visited Britain in 1982, the liberation front simply assumed that every Namibian female student on a scholarship in the country would be sexually available to the leaders. In Africa, radical student leaders boasted that they ruled their university campuses not just politically, but sexually too.

This brings us to hypothesis four: AIDS is a disease of patriarchy. At an individual level, gross inequalities in power between men and women and girls created sharp contours of risk of HIV. Desperately poor young women and girls traded their bodies for money. The terms 'commercial sex' and 'transactional sex' don't do justice to instances in which teenage girls were ready to exchange their first sexual encounters for the equivalent of a dollar or two, or for a snack and a drink. Many got HIV that way. This means that women are infected on average at a much younger age than men, and at higher levels too. That wouldn't happen if the girls were in school, with their school fees paid, lunch in their backpacks, looking forward to jobs after graduating. Gender inequality is a bad thing in itself, and HIV makes those power relations lethal. Women can rarely negotiate safe sex with their husbands and boyfriends, and in fact *not* using a condom is often a sign of trust in a relationship, even when each partner knows that the other has other concurrent sexual partners. Sex workers are often denigrated as a reservoir of HIV. But careful modelling of HIV risks shows that it is the men who control sex work who are the principal vector for introducing the virus into sex worker groups.[56] Experience of successful HIV prevention in the context of sex work also shows that what's most important is changing the behaviour of the pimps, brothel owners, and police – both their own sexual practices and whether or not they insist on clients using condoms.[57] None of these gender inequalities are unique to southern and eastern Africa, and in fact the status of women is even worse in other countries in Africa and in countries such as Yemen and Pakistan where HIV levels are low. In fact, at the very highest level of generalization, there is no correlation between gender inequality and HIV prevalence.[58] What is important for HIV is the way in which gendered power is an integral part of the sexual transactions web which is so efficient at spreading the virus.

Africa also has concentrated epidemics similar to those found elsewhere in the world: among men who have sex with men, intravenous drug users, sex workers and their clients, and patients who have been infected through contaminated needles or blood supplies.[59] These qualify as public health emergencies in their own right, but their numbers are hard to see amid the vast burden of the generalized epidemic.

The explanation for hyper-endemic HIV in southern and eastern Africa isn't a single factor, it's how all these elements came together. The colonial labour model and gender inequalities created a human landscape ideally suited for HIV, so that with the end of Apartheid, the end of armed conflict, and the end of austerity, there was greater mobility and there were increasing economic opportunities – and HIV. In Africa, AIDS was a disease of liberation shaped by a history of oppression. That's a characterization that resonates with the gay community in America and Europe.

Love and Liberation

AIDS brought with it an epidemic of moralizing, stereotyping, and fear-mongering. It also led to the most unexpected revolution in public health history. American gay men knocked down the gates of the citadel of the medical establishment and others – including international health officials and African activists – followed.

Almost exactly a hundred years after the investiture of Robert Koch in Berlin in May 1884, when the German kaiser announced the imminent conquest of cholera, the US Department of Health and Human Services held a press conference in Washington, DC. On 23 April 1984, Secretary Margaret Heckler announced that Robert Gallo had identified the retrovirus that caused AIDS.[60] Gallo named it human T-lymphotropic virus type III (HTLV-III, so numbered because he had previously isolated types I and II in his cancer research). Speaking softly because she was suffering laryngitis at the time, Heckler said:

> Today, I am pleased to . . . whisper that . . . the arrow of funds, medical expertise, research and experimentation with the Department of Health and Human Services, and its

allies around the world, have aimed and fired at the disease AIDS, and has hit the target only two or three rings away from the bullseye itself.

She explained that a test for the virus meant that it would be possible to screen blood donations and ensure that haemophiliacs were no longer at risk. Most of the press conference was taken up with the expected magic bullet – a vaccine – and how long it would take. It speaks to the power of the medical catechism that nobody asked the 'if' question, only the 'when'. One journalist mentioned the French scientist Luc Montagnier of the Pasteur Institute, who had identified what he called lymphadenopathy-associated virus (LAV) a year earlier and predicted that a vaccine would take five to ten years. Heckler's deputy Ed Brandt and Gallo said they were more 'optimistic': it could be done in two years or, at most, three. Unlike Kaiser Wilhelm, who had denounced the French, Heckler merely ignored Montagnier. Gallo denied that there had been 'any fights or controversies between us and a group in France'. This wasn't true: the dispute over who discovered the virus first was already acrimonious and became more so. In fact it needed a meeting between President François Mitterrand and President Ronald Reagan to reach a compromise that shared the honours – and to agree on the name HIV. More than 35 years on, the scrupulously technical name has stuck, and it is now the optimists who hope for a vaccine in five to ten years.

The military metaphors were routine, but political leaders were shy to use them. A disease afflicting stigmatized minorities didn't warrant putting the nation on a war footing. Reagan didn't mention AIDS at all for another 18 months, and only made his first speeches on the disease in 1987 when he attended a Hollywood fundraiser for the American Foundation for AIDS Research, after being implored by his old friend Elizabeth Taylor.

Talk of a vaccine raised the hopes of the most articulate and energetic constituency of affected people: gay men. A test for the virus meant that individuals could know their status. But HIV testing also opened up a scenario of surveillance, suppression, and control. Ever since the plague, states have enforced restrictions on citizens' rights in the name of public health. The celebrated case of 'Typhoid Mary' in New York in the early 20th century – the hapless woman who was a symptomless carrier of typhoid, spreading infection wherever she worked – was a test of whether the authorities had the power to incarcerate an individual who had committed no crime but who was a danger to public health. They did have that power, and human rights law has not disputed the principle. When AIDS was recognized, many countries quickly adopted regulations that restricted rights of movement and employment to people who were HIV-positive. Notably, the United States banned HIV-positive non-citizens from entry.[61] However, the wider feared crackdown didn't happen. To the contrary, in many places, AIDS became the occasion for more democratic and inclusive politics, and for some progress (modest, uneven) in recognizing the rights of sex workers, gay men, transsexuals, and survivors of rape.

For gay men, it was a fight for their lives, and a continuation of their struggle for rights and freedoms. More than anything else, it was the activism of gay men that made AIDS exceptional and created an entirely new model of emancipatory public health.[62] They challenged denial and discrimination. They insisted that people living with HIV and AIDS be involved in designing policies. They compelled the CDC and National Institutes of Health to listen to the demands of people affected by disease. They forced change in the protocols for research and testing for new medicines to recognize that for people suffering a life-threatening disease, the calculation of risk was very different to that of a government technocracy. In due course, they shamed the pharmaceutical corporations into bringing down the prices of drugs for treating AIDS. Together with activist health ministries in Brazil, India, and Thailand, the humanitarian agency Médecins Sans Frontières, and South African activists, they succeeded in making anti-retroviral therapy (ART) affordable in even the poorest countries. AIDS activists found allies in international organizations, first Jonathan Mann at the WHO's Global Programme on AIDS and then Peter Piot at UNAIDS.[63] Collectively, their single biggest achievement was what *didn't* happen: the pandemic of an incurable sexually transmitted disease didn't lead to a conservative moralistic counter-revolution and it wasn't the pretext for xenophobia or intrusive surveillance of people's private lives. All the criticisms of the international AIDS response have to be seen in the light of this achievement.

The biggest challenge for AIDS activism was in sub-Saharan Africa. Here, it encountered not only the biggest and most complex epidemic, but also conservative public sexual morality and enduring distrust of colonial medicine. The recycling of old 'heart of darkness' tropes and stories about African sexuality stoked further suspicion; the French acronym for the disease, SIDA, was satirized as *syndrome imaginaire pour décourager les amoureux* (imaginary syndrome to discourage lovers).

Where activism found an unexpected ally was in the revolutionary tradition of people's health, which had a lineage from China (barefoot doctors) and Cuba (Che Guevara's 'revolutionary medicine') to the African liberation struggle. An exemplar of this is Samora Machel, a nurse and leader of the Mozambican Liberation Front (Frelimo), who made people's health an integral part of the day-to-day practice of the people's war against Portuguese colonialism. In a speech to Frelimo cadres and foreign visitors in 1971, in the middle of the war, he contrasted the capitalist and colonialist hospital, which served to exploit people, with Frelimo's philosophy of people's health: 'Our hospitals belong to the people. They are a fruit of the revolution. Our hospitals are far more than centres for dispensing medicines and cures. A Frelimo hospital is a centre where our political line – that of serving the masses – is put into practice.' Frelimo's health workers were educators and political commissars. Machel concluded his speech: '[W]e define a Frelimo hospital as one of our fighting detachments, a front line.'[64]

Mozambicans fought to liberate themselves from the colonial occupier and from poverty, ignorance, and disease. At exactly that time, when Yoweri Museveni was a student at the University of Dar es Salaam and chair of the University Students African Revolutionary Front, he led a delegation to the liberated areas of Mozambique to support Frelimo, where his mentor and commander was Machel. There's a connection to AIDS. In 1986, Museveni attended his first summit of the Organization of African Unity (OAU) as Ugandan leader. He surprised his aides de camp by snapping to attention in the entrance to Africa Hall in Addis Ababa to salute his former commander, Machel (who was attending for the last time, as he was killed in a suspicious plane crash later in the year). At that same summit, Fidel Castro took Museveni aside to advise him, 'You know there is a big problem in your country.' Eighteen of the 60 Ugandan officers sent to Cuba for military training had tested HIV-positive.[65] It's likely that this was what prompted Museveni to start speaking candidly about AIDS.

When Africans of the liberation generation speak about 'war' against disease, their reference is liberation struggle. Thus, the veteran liberation leader and Secretary General of the OAU Salim Ahmed Salim opened an African conference on AIDS by saying, 'Our societies, in their entirety, have to enter into a combat mode for liberating themselves from the pandemic.'[66] Other African leaders joined in the fighting talk, including the UN Secretary General Kofi Annan, who called for a 'war chest' to fund AIDS efforts – which a year later became the Global Fund *to Fight* AIDS, Tuberculosis, and Malaria.

In Africa, HIV is overwhelmingly a sexually transmitted infection. As a rule, political leaders and senior officials in international organizations don't mention sex in public except to moralize and condemn. The talk about 'fighting'

AIDS was a way of *not* talking about sex. Graça Machel – an actual liberation fighter and educator and Samora's widow – preferred to use that platform to talk about the need for respecting and involving women and girls and changing men's values. She spoke about how liberation from oppression was not just overthrowing the oppressor but also creating a new sense of dignity. Machel also spoke about who had sex with whom and why: 'Some of our communities continue to educate young men with notions of manhood that encourage them viewing having multiple partners as natural and normal. . . . In this era of HIV/AIDS, different priorities must be developed and different values exemplified by our young men.'[67]

The moral energy of liberation can be fleeting but it can also be transformational. When first alerted to Uganda's AIDS problem, and still full of revolutionary fervour, Museveni authorized Africa's most candid public education programme. The main slogan was 'A, B, C' for 'Abstain, Be faithful, and use a Condom'. Specific messages were more creative. One was 'love carefully', which is a frank admission that there's not much point in preaching abstinence only. Another was 'zero grazing', which refers to a goat or cow tethered to a post so that it eats in one spot and doesn't roam around. This is a nicely precise metaphor for the problem of concurrent sexual partnerships. Speaking to girls in an elite secondary school, Museveni even told them that when they eat sweets they should keep the wrappers on.[68] This was the context for Lutaaya's 'Alone and Frightened'.

Most of those who practise armed liberation become addicted to the arms, not the liberation. Over the years, Museveni's reputation has been corroded by corruption, repression, and militarism. His wars became brutal operations of organized theft and atrocity; his idealistic young liberation fighters grew up to become brigands. Confident that war was an extension of their politics, they found that their politics was little more than coercion. So too with Africa's 'war' on AIDS: its instruments became co-opted

into the politics of raising resources and dispensing patronage. Museveni himself is a prime example of this. His early
energy and frankness in confronting AIDS earned him
favoured status among aid donors, and Uganda's budget
swelled accordingly. Later, when the George W. Bush
administration oriented its AIDS policies to conform with
the values of its Christian supporters, Museveni sang a new
song. He and his wife Janet – who had become an evangeli-
cal Christian – retold the story of AIDS policy in Uganda
as promoting conservative family values, which simply isn't
true. He became fiercely homophobic. And as anti-retroviral
drugs became available, Museveni wielded a new power of
patronage. One doctor who had worked with the army said,
'[I]f one sees the list of beneficiaries of Museveni's authoriza-
tion for treatment, it becomes difficult to avoid accusing him
of nepotism.'[69]

More than Museveni, more than Lutaaya, the face of
AIDS in Uganda was changed by the everyday activism of
women. They cared for children orphaned by AIDS, tended
to the sick, taught their children, organized their churches
and schools, and demanded more from the authorities.
Many were themselves living with HIV and AIDS. Richard
Dowden calls them the 'positive HIV-positive women'.[70]
The same story was repeated, everywhere, across Africa.

All activism is local, and the epidemics of HIV differ
according to the main modes of transmission, the community affected, and the political context. Those working in
the international AIDS response first developed a mantra,
'know your epidemic, know your response', and then added
'act on its politics'.[71] So too the general principles of challenging denial, stigma, and discrimination were adapted by
AIDS activists to their local circumstances. When they met
together, for example at the regular international HIV/AIDS
conferences, they shared a rhetoric that the disease was the
most important thing in the world, and that it mattered
politically because it *should* matter. But, when returning
home, every AIDS activist well knew that this wouldn't

work in their particular case. For AIDS activism to work, it needed local strategies, and in most cases that meant tying it to other issues that animated national politics. Even in countries where more than half of young adults could expect to contract HIV in their lifetimes, repeated public opinion surveys found that AIDS wasn't at the top of voters' lists of concerns.[72]

A fine example of this is the strategy of South Africa's Treatment Action Campaign (TAC) to demand that President Thabo Mbeki take AIDS seriously. Following Nelson Mandela as the second post-Apartheid president, Mbeki promised to transform the economy to benefit the disadvantaged majority – but he was also an AIDS denialist. Mbeki refused to believe that HIV caused AIDS and insisted that anti-retrovirals were toxic drugs promoted by pharmaceutical companies for their profits. Zackie Achmat, a veteran of the ANC and a gay man living with HIV, led TAC. He used many of the tactics from the anti-Apartheid struggle to protest against Mbeki's fatal inaction.[73] TAC mounted legal challenges that accused Mbeki and his health minister of being complicit in the deaths of millions. But Achmat, along with most of the TAC activists, was still an ANC supporter despite this. They saw Mbeki's government as *their* government; they wanted reform and not revolution. The activist strategy was to couple the demand for treatment to other progressive reforms, such as basic services (electricity, mains water supplies, public transport) for the country's under-provided townships alongside universal child support payments and a living wage. The Mandela–Mbeki ANC was still the embodiment of hope and change, and TAC wanted to be part of it. Some activists argued that AIDS was so exceptional, and Mbeki's denialism so egregious, that they shouldn't dilute their agenda; Achmat countered that AIDS was here to stay and that their campaign would only have the stamina to persist if it joined itself to the everyday demands of the majority. In a way, TAC was normalizing AIDS activism within routine politics, just as HIV had normalized itself in the communities. The measure of this strategy was that Mbeki was re-elected in 2004 without losing votes, but in time TAC achieved its goals too.

There were (and are) many failings and shortcomings in the global AIDS response.[74] There were many misplaced priorities and wasted funds, and metrics of 'success' became tied in to spending money and aligning policy documents rather than measuring real outcomes. Every aid institution managed to couple its own priority with AIDS, so that programmes ostensibly about HIV and AIDS were primarily funding education or agriculture or an unending circuit of workshops, conferences, and training sessions. The people who should have been the highest priority – such as drug users and sex workers – often found themselves at the end of the queue for attention, money, and rights. Essential progress on women's reproductive rights and on harm reduction programmes for injecting drug users have often been blocked by conservative governments, notably the United States. The elaborate infrastructure for AIDS meant that other health needs such as malaria and maternal health were squeezed. Activists became co-opted into a well-funded international bureaucracy. UNAIDS, which had done so much to put the disease on the international agenda, became trapped in this system too. And as soon as ART was provided at scale, the global AIDS campaign began to lose its energy, so that some of the longer-term unresolved questions were not addressed: how would the expanding cost of providing treatment be met? How would the next generation of ART be developed when HIV developed resistance to the current drugs? Most quickly and equally alarmingly, HIV's partner in parasitism and pillage, tuberculosis, has already evolved multi-drug-resistant strains which we can't treat: we can only sequester the people who have them in old-fashioned isolation hospitals. Antibiotic resistance is a spectrum of crises in waiting, and one of these crises is that it will turn our species' current condition of 'living with HIV' into an unending race to keep ahead of microbial evolution.

AIDS in the Margins of Error

Another catastrophe didn't happen. AIDS was expected to stoke global insecurity and, in the African countries where it was becoming hyper-endemic, to tear down the pillars of society. This is Whiteside's third wave: 'impact', which can't be represented with the same kind of quantitative precision, but which rears up behind the curve of AIDS deaths. What was going to happen to society when the wave of illness and death crashed ashore? What was AIDS's pandemy?

The scale of Africa's AIDS pandemic became clear at the same time as the US national security establishment was in turmoil. It had won its biggest ever victory quite unexpectedly, and that posed a problem. Its Cold War enemy had disappeared and politicians were asking whether the entire military-industrial and security-intelligence apparatuses served any purpose other than a costly employment generation scheme. America's triumph ranked among the worst failures in the annals of intelligence history: busy counting missiles, it hadn't foreseen the collapse of the Soviet Union. Just one small group of analysts stood out: health statisticians. In the 1970s, Christopher Davis (Britain's leading academic on Soviet public health) and Murray Feshbach (the US Census Bureau's expert on Soviet demography) looked at the figures for infant mortality in the USSR and saw that they were rising. After some debate over whether the figures were in fact accurate (they were), the two published a short, dispassionate, and devastating summary.[75] Nick Eberstadt, then a young academic embarking on a career in political science, reviewed the findings and argued that something was going wrong not just with the Soviet health care system, but with the economy as a whole.[76] The fact that every indicator for the health of the ordinary people of the USSR was pointing downwards showed, he said, that the Soviet system wasn't sustainable. Communism's social contract was unravelling. At this point, Eberstadt's prognosis went off course:

he suggested that an adventurist Soviet leadership might provoke an international crisis to make up for its domestic economic failures and didn't consider the possibility that Communist rule would crumble from within.[77] All the same, the experts who dealt with health metrics emerged from the shambles of security forecasting in Washington, DC, in 1989–91 with their reputation enhanced.

Demographers' standing got another boost when the post-Cold War era began to look like a slide into anarchy. Nineteen ninety-four was the nadir year: protracted war in former Yugoslavia, imbroglio for the UN in Cambodia, humiliating US withdrawal from Somalia, a rogue dictatorship defying American pressure in Haiti, and genocide in Rwanda. President Bill Clinton read Kaplan's 'Coming Anarchy' article and instructed that it be faxed to every US embassy around the world. Vice President Al Gore instructed the CIA to convene a 'State Failure Task Force' drawing on leading academics to figure out which countries were most at risk of descent into chaos. It was an exercise in massive political science number crunching, throwing every possible variable or indicator into the analytical pot to see what came out. When the Task Force processed its data to generate the best models for predicting state failure, it found three variables from among its list of 75 to be the most important: openness to trade, democracy, and infant mortality.[78]

They didn't claim that young children dying would directly cause revolutions, civil wars, or the disintegration of government institutions. As statisticians insist, causation isn't correlation. But their data showed that this correlation wasn't just back in the USSR – it held true around the world. Health wasn't just about health, it was about national security too. Many public health leaders welcomed the language of security because it opened the door to the corridors of power and promised money from security budget lines.[79] Conventional security analysts – as soon as they had regained their footing after the tremors of 1989 – generally didn't consider health (nor, for that matter, climate and poverty) as a 'real' security issue. Soldiers were becoming embroiled in 'new wars' that involved irregular soldiers and criminal gangs, waged for profit or ethnic bigotry, which threatened to go on indefinitely,[80] and disease was part of this Hobbesian 'warre' against which they were fighting. They considered 'human security' talk to be soft and the idea that soldiers might 'fight' disease (or poverty, illiteracy, or climate change) a distraction. Reluctantly, health and security were locked in the same policy room and had to find a way to get along.

Their agreed starting point was that soldiers were at risk from the virus. Men in uniform get sexually transmitted diseases. A worrying number of recruits in eastern Europe and the former Soviet Union contracted HIV through injecting drug use and the Russian military feared that, combined with tuberculosis and alcoholism, there might not be enough healthy young men for military service. The UN Department of Peacekeeping Operations was trying to work out how to manage the countries that contributed peacekeepers (each of which had its own distinct national policy), the countries where they were deployed (which didn't want them bringing in HIV), and the UN's paymasters (who wanted the highest standards for policies). Western countries that were deploying their own troops on humanitarian missions to Africa and Haiti were concerned that those soldiers might get infected.

Worse, intelligence analysts began to make the case that the AIDS pandemic would cause massive social disruption and state failure. The CIA reported on this as early as 1987.[81] In 1996, a presidential decision directive identified infectious diseases as a threat to national and international security. It was introduced by Health and Human Services Secretary Donna Shalala with these words: 'The Clinton Administration has made the war against emerging infectious diseases a priority. . . . These diseases know no boundaries, and our international pursuit of them must know no end.'[82] The US National Intelligence Council compiled a report on infectious diseases as a national security threat.[83] Gore worked with the head of UNAIDS, Peter Piot, and a small coterie of diplomats over the Christmas break in 1999 to spring a New Year surprise: the UN Security Council's first meeting of the millennium was on infectious diseases as a threat to international peace and security. They pulled it off because China and Russia didn't have fully staffed embassies in place over the holiday season. Those countries, with more traditional views on health and security, accepted a discussion and a statement, but not a resolution – when that came, later in 2000, it focused on UN peacekeeping only. Some analysts at the CIA and their public health counterparts were concerned that the biggest danger was a 'next wave' of HIV that would generate new epicentres in China, India, and Russia, with those countries following the southern African trajectory towards generalized epidemics.[84]

The most immediate concern was sub-Saharan Africa, where HIV rates were truly scary: Botswana and Swaziland surpassed 30 per cent prevalence among adults and South Africa was close behind. Life expectancy dropped from over 60 years to about 45. And those figures didn't really capture the gravity of the problem. The conventionally used figure – life expectancy at birth – understated the crisis, because AIDS kills adults in their twenties, thirties, and forties, unlike the customary pattern of mortality in a poor country, which is a high rate of infant and child deaths and a relatively healthy adulthood. In a population without ART, HIV prevalence rates translate to lifetime chances of contracting HIV in a ratio of one to three-to-five: that is, with a 10 per cent HIV prevalence in the adult population, a young person has between a 30 and a 50 per cent chance of contracting the virus during her or his lifetime.[85] With a 25 per cent prevalence, getting AIDS approaches statistical certainty. To put it another way, a high-school graduate in Europe or America can expect 40 to 50 years of working life, followed by retirement; she can look forward to seeing her grandchildren graduate too. Across southern Africa, life expectancy at 20 had dropped to about 25 more years.[86] A 20-year-old woman could expect two decades of active adult life followed by AIDS. No mature adulthood with grown-up children; no financially stable home; no fulfilling career. In turn it would no longer make economic sense for governments and corporations to invest in further education and training, as too many of their staff would die before they could put their skills to use.

By contrast, the 1918 influenza cut life expectancy around the world by 10 years during just one year, after which it rebounded. Great famines cut life expectancy more deeply, but transiently in the stricken countries. A sustained halving of adult lifespans had never been experienced since the great plagues 650 years ago. The kind of existential threat faced by gay men and injecting drug users was being replicated at the scale of half a continent. Researchers began the frightening process of exploring what this meant, asking whether the basic institutions of society could still function under these medieval life chances. I was among them. They (we) wrote about HIV/AIDS causing 'development in reverse'; creating a generation of unschooled and poorly socialized orphans; eviscerating armies and police forces; combining with war in a vicious cycle of despair and decay; and sparking violent protests and bloody revolutions. Alan Whiteside and I proposed that it would drive 'new variant famine' and that it would 'hollow out' institutions, putting state-building into reverse gear.[87]

None of the predictions came true. To be more exact, there were many dreadful impacts, but Africa didn't collapse. Over the following 10 years, African economies grew; democracy expanded; and the continent's institutions became stronger. In the early 2000s, when the predictions were at their most frightening, I helped initiate three research exercises into the likely impacts of HIV and AIDS. These were the UN Commission on HIV/AIDS and Governance in Africa, the HIV/AIDS, Conflict, and Security Initiative, and the Joint Learning Initiative on Children and HIV/AIDS (the second two covering not just Africa but the world).[88] By the time each of them reported in 2008–9, they described how and why things *hadn't* collapsed, in Africa and elsewhere in the world. Neither international agencies such as UNAIDS, nor researchers, are good at examining why they got their analyses wrong – especially when bad things that were forecast didn't happen – but the reasons why we got them wrong are important and fascinating.

The most straightforward reason is that the epidemic curve for AIDS illness and death didn't follow the projections because of ART. Not only did treatment stop people from dying, but it also lifted fear and stigma. Between them, the Global Fund to Fight AIDS, Tuberculosis, and Malaria and the President's Emergency Plan for AIDS Relief (PEPFAR) provided treatment to millions. An equally big part of the reason why the worst outcomes were averted was that the rate of infection was slowing even before ART became available. The best evidence for this is to compare the epidemiological projections for HIV with what actually happened. The models couldn't take account of how people's behaviour changed. If we construct a model that can be retrofitted to the epidemic curve as it actually unfolded, the key factors are elements such as older age of first sex for young women, and fewer concurrent sexual partners, which happened regardless of official policies and type of government. HIV levels came down in Zimbabwe (bankrupt, repressive, and strife-riven), and in South Africa (which had an AIDS denialist for president during the crucial years), just as they did in Uganda (widely acclaimed for its AIDS policies) and in Ethiopia (which had an exemplary programme run by a health minister whose record was the basis for his later elevation to head the WHO). In short, the epidemic didn't turn out to be quite as horrendous as anticipated. But even with a somewhat flattened curve, the disease was still far worse than anything the continent had experienced since pandemic influenza, and that should have caused terrible social and political outcomes as well as numberless personal tragedies.

In retrospect, the model for how African societies worked was too simple and in many respects simply wrong. There were two big errors in thinking about 'developing' countries, and especially 'failed' and 'fragile' states. First, the State Failure Task Force, and every subsequent exercise at constructing a worldwide index, ranked countries in a league table from the most functional (emblematically, Denmark) to the least (Somalia, Afghanistan, and Liberia vied for the bottom spot). Countries gained or lost points for their scores on variables such as armed conflict, democracy, foreign investment, life expectancy, and so on. This implies that good things (rule of law, prosperity, etc.) go together, and conversely that bad things (war, corruption, disease) also go together and make one another worse. These assessments are implicit in words such as 'developing country' and 'failed state'. Those who construct these indices are aware of this simplification, but ignore it for practical purposes, partly because of the reinforcement they get from institutions such as the World Bank that use them. Moreover, the positive correlation between indicators holds up in a general manner, because violence harms people and societies.[89] But the link doesn't necessarily hold for a specific infectious disease, and it turned out not to be true that HIV and AIDS interacted with other bad things, stacking on top of one another. For example, contrary to what we expected, war and HIV didn't go together, and neither were HIV rates associated with cuts in GDP per capita. Discomforting though it was to those of us with humane sensibilities, higher death rates *increased* GDP per capita by reducing the denominator (population) more than the enumerator (output).[90]

Another implication is that a weak (developing, fragile, failed) state is in a relegation spot because it lacks something that the better performers have, namely institutions. Here we must be aware of a mental sleight of hand. Try a Google Images search for 'institution' and the algorithm delivers icons of classical buildings with columns and porticos.[91] We think of an institution as a solid and enduring physical establishment housing a legal-rational and impersonal bureaucracy. With its disturbing ability to pre-empt our thought processes, Google Images selects pictures with grand buildings where human beings are small and transient. Now turn to a search for the academic definition of 'institution' and it becomes clear that the everyday use of a word can be different to its specialist social scientific use. From Max Weber onwards, social scientists have defined 'institutions' as established social practices. For example, the influential political science theorist Douglass North defines institutions as 'the humanly devised constraints that structure political, economic, and social interaction. They consist of both informal constraints (sanctions, taboos, customs, traditions, and codes of conduct), and formal rules (constitutions, laws, property rights).'[92] An everyday version of this is in 'the institution of marriage'. A common mistake made by students and policymakers, such as the officials of aid organizations working to reconstruct conflict-ravaged countries, is to assume that these kinds of 'social norm institutions' *ought* to resemble the formal legal-rational bureaucracies of Protestant nations in north-west Europe and North America, and that anything that doesn't is somehow deficient.

Examined closely, the AIDS crisis in Africa showed how 'norm institutions' were more important than formal institutions. This can be shown by returning to look at what 'hollowing out' means for two different kinds of institutions. The models assumed that the labour, skill, and experience of adults were needed to keep formal institutions functioning, to keep economies productive, and to import social norms to the next generation. It seems not.

Take the case of armies, perhaps the simplest case. The worry that animated both traditional security analysts and the human security people was that illness and death among the officer corps would strip armies of the experience and expertise they needed and leave them as undisciplined wrecks. What happened was that, despite AIDS afflicting officers, armies continued to function. What was rediscovered was that armies are designed to operate even while soldiers die. They have built-in redundancy, which should have been obvious because an army fighting a war expects to suffer casualties. Something comparable held for civil institutions and corporations. We face the troubling fact that human capital isn't needed as much as we thought; a lot of human knowledge and skill is superfluous to social and economic need, and enormous suffering doesn't necessarily cause social crisis.

Recall that sub-Saharan Africa had recently endured an economic recession that was so deep that it had called into question the viability of basic governmental functioning. This wasn't just a setback to be endured on the road to development, it was a test of social and political survival skills, from which African people and their leaders emerged having learned some tough lessons. Politicians who had managed to hang on to power, seeing off the challenges of armed rivals, applied the skills of the wheeler-dealer to the business of politics. Africanist political scientists described the hybrid of formal government apparatus and informal patronage systems as 'neo-patrimonial'; I prefer to describe it as a political marketplace in a state of continual turbulence in which those most adept at adapting to unpredictable market conditions are most likely to survive.[93] The members of the new African political elite tacitly recognize the mercenary rules whereby political allegiances and services are bought and sold. They can shape formal institutions to resemble templates from donor countries, for the purposes of obtaining funds and achieving some important shared goals, but they actually run them with patronage and graft. Transactional politics trumped legal-bureaucratic rationality. It wasn't the performance of these formal institutions according to public metrics of success that made African governments resilient, it was skill in operating the transactional networks of 'real politics'.

Transactional politics is, in itself, value neutral: it can be bent towards kleptocratic autocratic dynasties, towards a collusive cartel of crony capitalists and securocrats, or towards progressive social change. Other African leaders, who had nurtured democracy movements while in exile or in prison, or who had kept their liberation movements intact through the years when things fell apart, recognized that Africa needed to revitalize its norms and principles. They set about reforming the OAU and building a new African continental organization based on collective responsibility for intervening to end atrocities, ostracizing coup makers, bringing peaceful settlements to wars, and presenting a common front of better governance to international donors. Behind the formal theatre of African Union summits, politicians bargained over political favours, but the pressure of their peers to keep up appearances gradually rewrote the rules of the political game to align with peace, democracy, and international cooperation. Building formal institutions for democracy, rule of law, and economic management was part of this, but what made these formal institutions matter was the informal understandings worked out in a web of political transactions. The fact that AIDS became a billion-dollar industry sent a message to this mercenary world where money is the most respected measure of value: AIDS counted. It was in everyone's interests to have a best-practice AIDS programme.

Africans had withstood the depredations of colonialism and the austerity and turmoil of the late-century crises, and expected few benefits from their states. As AIDS unfolded, those unmeasured and unrecognized capacities for coping and caring again served their purpose. There were millions of children orphaned by AIDS, but no bands of unsocialized vagrants. Extended families took care of almost all of them. And, as a general phenomenon, Africa's young and fast-growing population simply meant that in every sector, there were energetic and keen young people filling the gaps. The dire forecasts for AIDS-related social crisis also didn't take into account the power of community mobilization and hope. Models are built on routines and rules, and when people change those, the models no longer apply.

No Singular Story

Activism changed everything. If there is an example of emancipatory pandemic response, the coalition that organized against AIDS is it. Peter Piot ends his memoir with a reflection on the practical value of shared moral outrage: 'The global response to AIDS was a rare exception to the iron rule that international aid is fundamentally an extension of foreign policy and foreign trade. . . . It is perhaps the strongest example of global altruism out of a rational necessity in our ever-more connected world.'[94] It's also the best example of how activism can change norms and narratives. For the most part, this was something to celebrate, but with time and money, the new way of thinking itself became institutionalized.

When AIDS was first identified in America and Europe, the key narrative was stigma, exclusion, and conservative moralizing. Gay men were blamed. They resisted in a vigorous way that articulated new models and storylines. They contested the martial script from the start. In 1988, Susan Sontag wrote, 'About that metaphor, the military one, give it back to the warmakers.'[95] It still hung around, however, like an unwanted guest who wouldn't take the hint. Programmes were established to 'fight' AIDS; vaccines and therapies were promised to 'defeat' it. When people became scared about AIDS in the military and AIDS and national security, they used the language of 'invisible enemy', but rarely with much verve or conviction. And in eastern and southern Africa, where AIDS was a truly existential threat, the 'war' narrative that resonated was liberation war – but that didn't go much beyond political rhetoric.

Policing AIDS was more crucial and revealing. For those who led the AIDS movement, the real fear – along with the disease – was that the virus would validate societal stigma and discrimination and legitimize intrusive governmental policing and surveillance. This didn't happen. Stigma and discrimination were persistent and pervasive, but it is astonishing how rarely they were formalized in official government policies. In fact, the neglect of police forces in HIV/AIDS policy and planning is quite remarkable, and is matched with a counterpart neglect of HIV by most police forces. It's a revealing blind spot. Many people at high risk of HIV come into close contact with the police, because they are at the margins of the law. Some act unlawfully, some are victims of crimes, many are in communities or contexts that are officially profiled as dangerous. Drug users, pimps and sex workers, people traffickers and their victims, survivors of sexual violence, prisoners, people with sexualities or gender identities that aren't socially approved – all of them are at higher risk of HIV and also have frequent interaction with the police. But when my colleague Jennifer Klot and I convened a meeting of police officers from around the world to discuss these topics in The Hague in 2007, we discovered that this was the first time this had been done.[96] The international AIDS business had overlooked the institution that literally policed the disease. The people who came to the meeting were chosen because they had innovated creative ways for police services to engage sympathetically with the issues of HIV and AIDS, or were police officers living with HIV, and all advocated for more and better police practices. We wanted more action. None of us reflected on the hidden virtues of neglect. If police forces had taken it upon themselves to police AIDS, they might have been repressive in a more systematic and draconian manner.

The global AIDS response became huge and institutionalized – in both senses of the word, as norms and bureaucracies. Like any such large institution, it began to take itself and its ways of thinking about the world for granted. Agencies like UNAIDS became like the inflexible institutions they had initially been set up to circumvent, stuck following their own narrative while the science moved on.

The virus didn't conform: HIV has a special genius of finding people who don't fit into bureaucratic categories. Lisa Pisani writes about her experience of conducting multiple-choice questionnaire surveys to find out who was at most risk of HIV. She takes the case of Fuad, an Indonesian 21-year-old who occasionally worked as a truck driver's assistant and who bought sex from a transgender 'waria':

> Fuad's girlfriend was doubtless a nice girl. She also worked the streets of Bandung at night. So here we have a self-proclaimed heterosexual guy who has unpaid sex with a woman who sells sex to other men, while himself also selling sex to other men and buying it from transgendered sex workers. He pushed a lot of the 'high risk' buttons for HIV infection, yet he wasn't a female sex worker, a client, a drug injector, a gay man or a student. He didn't fit into a single one of our questionnaire boxes. The truth is, real people don't have sex in boxes.[97]

Pisani spent years trying to make UNAIDS realign its policies to accord with discomforting evidence such as this. She found it harder and harder as time went on. Liberal institutions have learned the skill of licensing dissent and then carrying on as before, and Pisani finally quit her job when her colleagues began anticipating her critiques and discounting them. She writes that it had become an institution 'where money eclipses truth'.[98]

The AIDS business constructed identity boxes that began by liberating people and ended up confining them. Early on, activists led the way in recognizing and celebrating identity groups that had been stigmatized. Female mobilization was the key to almost every success in sub-Saharan Africa and progress was made in lockstep with improving the rights and well-being of women and girls – an unmitigated good. But some successes left radicals uncomfortable with what they had won. Gay rights activists brought their agenda home into the political mainstream with the campaign for gay marriage.[99] Conservative Christians switched from seeing AIDS as punishment of the wicked to an affliction of the innocent, which contributed to President Bush's setting up PEPFAR with its additional agenda of restricting reproductive rights and banning abortion. Each time the activists gained ground they found many others moving in to occupy it. That is the tribute that conservatives pay to social change, the ambiguous index of progress in equality and emancipation.

Emancipatory public health didn't 'defeat' HIV and AIDS. But in partnership with biomedical science it changed society so that we can manage AIDS and cohabit with endemic HIV. It's too early to write even the first draft of the obituary of HIV and AIDS: the current regimen is a temporary parity between biomedical progress and viral evolution. Maintaining that parity depends upon continued activism and continued pharmaceutical research and drug development. There isn't a singular regime of truth for HIV and AIDS, as Michel Foucault might have concluded, had he not died from the disease in 1984. Or at least, there's no orderly narrative. In response to the pandemic, affected people and activist public health officials tried out diverse new narratives. They achieved a lot: in their day-to-day frustrations it is easy to forget how much has been achieved, and how much worse things could have been. The biggest achievement was mobilizing people for social change. If one of the many dramatists who succumbed to AIDS were to write a script for this story, they could conclude by adapting the final scene of Brecht's *Threepenny Opera*, in which the house lights are turned on and the audience become protagonists, not spectators.[100]

5

Imagined Unknowns: Pandemic X

Pathogen X is the feared germ that generates Pandemic X. It doesn't exist, at least not yet. In the previous chapters, I have anthropomorphized the microbes as a guide to understanding their logics. Pathogen X is different: it's solely a work of human imagination. Analysing it makes clear our hopes, fears, and narratives. That makes it easier to describe. It can't disrupt our paradigms because it *is* a paradigm.

Ebola was the first suspect for Pathogen X. The virus was known, but not where it came from and what it might do. As recently as 2006, the reservoir for Ebola remained a puzzle: was it rodents, bats, arthropods, or even plants? Researchers thought that indications of Ebola virus RNA and antibodies in bats were 'intriguing' and 'promising'.[1] We now know that bats are a reservoir for many viruses including Ebola, and that zoonotic jumps are becoming more common as bats' habitats are disrupted and they come into more regular contact with humans.

Ebola is a filovirus, so called because under the electron microscope it looks like a string (Latin *filum* = thread) with a loop at one end. When it infects a human, the first symptoms are like flu, followed by diarrhoea, vomiting, and

internal bleeding. In severe cases, the virus goes on to replicate at a prodigious rate, turning internal organs into viral
stew, causing massive bleeding internally and from every ori-
fice, including the eyes. It's about as lethal as the plague in
the 14th century or cholera in the mid-19th century. There
are several strains of filovirus, including Ebola's close cousin
Marburg virus, named after the German town where there
was an outbreak that began with monkeys imported from
Uganda. There were simultaneous (but unrelated) outbreaks
of Ebola in 1976, in the town of Maridi in southern Sudan
(now the independent country of South Sudan), and at the
Yambuku mission in Zaïre (now the Democratic Republic
of Congo). Ebola-Sudan killed about half of those infected
(151 deaths from 284 confirmed cases). Ebola-Zaïre killed
nearly 90 per cent (280 deaths from 318). In a peculiarly
tragic turn, as we will discuss later in this chapter, the nurses
and nuns at the Yambuku mission were unwitting agents of
infection because they reused just a handful of needles for
numerous injections of pregnant women with vitamin shots,
rinsing them with warm water between each use and only
sterilizing them overnight. Because the disease progresses
rapidly, outbreaks in isolated communities usually kill so
quickly that the virus doesn't travel far, like a bushfire that
blazes fiercely but in a confined area on a windless day. The
two 1976 outbreaks remained the largest by far until 2014,
and most outbreaks killed a dozen or so. There was, at the
time, neither vaccine nor cure.

Monkeys can also be infected. In 1989, a monkey captured
in the Philippines and shipped to America for laboratory
research brought with it a novel strain of Ebola. Monkeys
held in a holding facility belonging to Hazelton Laboratories
at Reston, Virginia, just off the road from Dulles Airport to
Washington, DC, started falling sick and dying. The outbreak was contained by the US army in an operation that
was kept quiet. This particular strain of Ebola had gained the
terrifying capability of becoming airborne: it was spread by
coughing, sneezing, and even through the ventilation system

of the warehouse where the monkeys were held. By good fortune, inexplicable to virologists, Ebola-Reston, though lethal in monkeys, didn't cause illness in humans. One monkey, smuggled out of a San Francisco port quarantine facility to be sold as a pet, harboured another respiratory strain which had the converse characteristic: the monkey was a symptomless carrier but the virus was lethal to humans. This new-variant filovirus caused an outbreak in a small Californian town and confronted US military and civilian health officials with an awful dilemma: destroy the community and the people who lived there, or risk the outbreak becoming pandemic.

Most of this actually happened – until the story of the smuggled monkey in California, which is fiction. The story of Ebola in Africa is told first-hand by Peter Piot, then a young researcher at the Antwerp Tropical Institute and a member of the team that isolated the virus. The American side of the origins story, followed by the outbreak at Reston, is told by the journalist Richard Preston in his book *The Hot Zone*.[2] From the smuggled monkey onwards, it is the plotline of the movie *Outbreak*.[3] There's a simple reason why the next rewrite of the 'war on disease' script was the work of novelists, movie directors, and simulation designers. The definitive pandemic of the turn of the millennium was the fearsome 'coming plague' that *hadn't happened yet*.[4]

For many years, specialists in emerging diseases spoke of the 'Big One' or the 'Next Big One', sometimes 'NBO'.[5] The virologist Edwin Kilbourne invented the 'maximally malignant (monster) virus', a hybrid of all the deadliest characteristics of known viruses – 'the environmental stability of poliovirus, the antigenic mutability of influenza virus, the unrestricted host range of rabies virus, and the latency or reactivation potential of a herpes virus' – complete with its own acronym, MMMV.[6] The one thing missing from the MMMV's lethal recipe was that it didn't possess a sociological sixth sense – it didn't utilize the most vital economic and social circuits for its transmission. The term 'Disease X' was formally adopted by the WHO in 2018 to make the point that governments around the world needed to be ready for the outbreak of an infectious agent new to medical science. Aerosolized Ebola is among the most potentially apocalyptic pathogens that meet these WHO criteria.[7] Because Outbreak X hadn't happened, and Pathogen X hadn't even been discovered, it could only be written as a scientifically plausible scenario – in short, as science fiction. It is a bit like the imagined monster of a horror movie, the drumbeat and dorsal fin of the unseen shark in *Jaws*, all the more horrific because its true character hasn't been revealed.

Preparing for Disease X is a task of creativity and rigour: the virologist has to imagine the possible character of the pathogen and the public health planner has to think of credible epidemiological scenarios. It's an exercise in trying to anticipate how wrong we might be. It's the task of doing just enough rethinking in advance that we won't have to do more fundamental rethinking when the worst happens. Simulation scenario designers for epidemics do their scientific homework on transmission patterns and disease virulence and then tweak the variables; they add in information about emergency health capacities and vaccine production times, and develop a plausible plotline about how people and governments will react. This is similar to the creative processes of science fiction writers, such as Michael Crichton (*The Andromeda Strain*) and Guillermo del Toro and Chuck Hogan (*The Strain*). It is also a version of alternative world-building that appeals to people who design video games, who create parallel realities in which most – but not all – of the rules of our own world apply. The reader or player recognizes these worlds at once, which are based on plotlines that follow well-rehearsed conventions of characterization and dramaturgy. As noted in chapter 1, if the author or designer is suspending one rule about reality, other rules should be held steady or the reader will become bewildered. The same constraints hold for the narrative arc of the imagined Pandemic X: it must be just familiar enough to be readily thinkable.

'Outbreak'

This chapter tells the following story. After the emergence of HIV, infectious disease specialists became worried about pathogens, known and unknown, with pandemic potential. There was a debate within this professional community and their specialist institutions, especially the WHO and the CDC. One challenge they faced was how to formulate uncertainty in a manner that was consistent with their scientifically honed intuitions and which could also resonate with senior government officials, who didn't possess that refined scientific literacy. They found allies among security analysts who had developed ways of thinking about and modelling uncertainties beyond readily calculable risk and presenting these in a manner that persuaded their political masters. In the 1990s, pandemic risk was an inconvenient truth that didn't get its political break. That changed in 2001 when bio-terrorism became a priority threat. The national security establishment and the infectious disease community found a common cause. Pandemic preparedness got lots of money and adopted a 'war on terror' model.

In her book *Contagious*, the literature professor Priscilla Wald dissects both fictional and factual storylines and diagnoses what she calls the 'outbreak narrative'.[8] She describes it as 'a formulaic plot that begins with the identification of an emerging infection, includes discussion of the global networks through which it travels, and chronicles the epidemiological work that ends with its containment'.[9] The 'outbreak narrative' comes in several strains. Ebola is the African jungle variant: the pathogen is an ancient predator lurking in the primaeval forest, infecting humans who have encroached on its domain. There is also an East Asian shanty town version. The killer sneaks out in an infected animal, or an unwitting tourist, businessperson, or researcher brings it into the midst of civilization. It's both a medical and a security emergency. The race is on. In their sealed hazmat suits, medical scientists seek a vaccine or a therapy, and military commanders organize a siege which they call bio-containment. In the fictional storyline, the intruder is defeated.[10] In the simulation, the scenario exercise doesn't have a happy ending: it stops with the invader out of control, as a warning to the participants that we are unprepared for this assault.

The outbreak narrative usually begins in the disrupted wildernesses of faraway countries. In *The Hot Zone*, Preston describes the virus hunter looking out of an aeroplane window over the African jungle with its snaking rivers, oxbow lakes, and mottled tree canopy, knowing that a mysterious microbe hides there, and also looking through the microscope at the landscape of human cells, as though scanning a terra incognita, seeking – and finding – the killer virus.[11] Preston writes of the 'heart of Africa'; he is just one literary step away from the heart of darkness, which is a step he doesn't take, but the reader knows that Joseph Conrad's novel was set in the same middle reaches of the Congo river.

Earlier drafts of the outbreak narrative classified some infectious diseases as foreign and extended the stigma to their human carriers as well. The contemporary script plays to this familiar association, though writers and movie makers carefully tread around overtly racist portrayals. The new version also introduces a secular version of an old theology: diseases break out because the world is out of kilter, because humans have disturbed a natural equilibrium. In some fictionalized versions, there's also a subplot of scientific hubris, such as the blowback from a bioweapons accident.

Because it's difficult to cast a microbe as a villain, fiction (especially film) needs human baddies. In the 1995 movie *Outbreak* (directed by Wolfgang Petersen), the human villain is Major General Donald McClintock (played by Donald Sutherland), who had encountered the virus in the 1960s but kept his knowledge secret to develop an illegal bioweapon, and also because he had firebombed a military camp to stop that jungle outbreak. The general wants to use the same method – obliteration – on the Californian town of Cedar Creek, until he is prevented at the last moment by the heroics of an army doctor, Colonel Sam Daniels (played by Dustin Hoffman), with civilian research scientist Roberta Keogh (played by Rene Russo), who develops a serum that cures the infected. It's a melodramatic denouement with a race between a miraculous medical cure and epidemic eradication by fuel-air explosives. Medicine wins over bombing but the audience is left wondering what would happen if no such magic bullet had been found.

Outbreak is Hollywood's dramatization of alarm bells pressed by Laurie Garrett and Richard Preston. They in turn wrote the popular versions of weighty reports compiled by infectious disease experts. The Ur-text is the 300-page *Emerging Infections* compiled by the Committee on Emerging Microbial Threats to Health at the US Institute of Medicine under the leadership of Joshua Lederberg.[12] This was the culmination of three years of research and conferences by the National Institutes of Health, the US National Academy of Sciences, and the WHO.[13] As well as HIV – which had been the wake-up call – the list of emerging diseases included Ebola and Marburg virus, Creutzfeldt–Jakob disease, Hantavirus, Lyme disease, and Zika virus. Some were resurgent old pathogens such as plague in India, cholera in Peru, and yellow fever in Kenya. Some were known diseases in new places such as dengue in South America, or Chikungunya and West Nile Fever, which were first identified in central Africa but were spreading elsewhere. A return of pandemic influenza, a rerun of 1918–19, was identified as the biggest danger. Creeping into the discussion was the possibility of a pandemic pathogen for which medical science and public health were wholly unprepared.

The committee first appraised America. Then in April 1994, Lederberg convened a meeting of experts from every continent at WHO headquarters in Geneva. Lederberg opened the meeting by referring to his book *Emerging Infections*, saying that while it 'was targeted to the United States, 70–80% of the issues were of global concern'. The memo from the meeting records a consensus from the discussion: 'Clearly a global approach, spearheaded by the World Health Organization, is needed to address the problem.'[14] Most of their action points involved matters such as linking clinical, epidemiological, and laboratory programmes around the world, better coordination of information, and new initiatives for vaccine development. They lamented the decay in public health infrastructure in most countries and bemoaned the lack of public awareness. To help close that last gap, Lederberg advised the movie *Outbreak*, and it opens with his words: 'The single biggest threat to man's continued dominance on this planet is the virus.'

Institutionalizing Uncertainty

In the previous chapter, I introduced an analysis of social institutions as shared mechanisms for regulating thinking. Norm institutions enable human societies to encode and process information and take decisions. To use another simile, institutions extract the salient and actionable signal from the noise. The concept of 'risk' is one way of classifying uncertainty by putting a number on some forms of uncertainty (those that can be measured) and deciding to ignore those forms that are incalculable. The insurance business distinguishes between everyday risks, for which its routine calculations can work out liabilities, and catastrophic risks, which don't submit to formulae and require government action such as a bail-out. The boundary between routine and calamitous risk is blurred and shifting. Advances in scientific knowledge make more risks calculable, while the rising tide of climate crisis is lifting all other perils.

Academic disciplines and policy communities are institutions *par excellence* and each has its own particular doctrines and instruments for risk and uncertainty. At one end of the spectrum, seismologists deal with events that are potentially catastrophic and (in the short term) very hard to predict.

Climate scientists grapple with the challenge of making their professional consensus about the catastrophic trajectory of global heating into a credible popular narrative that acknowledges uncertainties in the data and models and generates the right combination of fear and hope among the public and politicians. At the other end, economists who are devoted to equilibrium theories are poorly equipped to understand calamities, including those, such as stock market crashes, that are generated by economic systems themselves. Sociologists and political scientists specialize at espying order where laypeople see chaos, and sometimes take their models too seriously for everyone's good. In each of these disciplines, it isn't just the internal debate that matters. Academics need to be validated by politicians, civil servants, and the media, and what gets approved is what gets funds, which shapes how scientific findings are presented to the public.

Public health policymakers and epidemiologists are spread across this spectrum of comfort or discomfort with uncertainty depending on what particular issue they study and how they think about it. Our concern here is not with cancer, obesity, or car safety, but with novel pandemic disease – exactly the kind of uncertainty that can't be calculated and is therefore excluded from the everyday calculus of risk. In the 18th century, mathematicians made transformative contributions to public health when they compiled the data for life expectancy and calculated the gains that would follow universal smallpox inoculation, but they couldn't predict the course of a new disease such as cholera. Today's virus-hunting microbiologist says that a novel pandemic is not actually uncertain at all, and that over time it is as close to a certainty as can exist in the world. That's the paradoxical epistemology of the epidemiology of pandemic preparedness. And, as with every other discipline, when the organized data aren't there, we write a storyline. At a personal level, that's the basis for narrative medicine, which helps patients, as people, understand the path of illness and recovery, or lack thereof.[15] Narrative medicine draws on a whole range of metaphors, such as journeying, schooling, fairground rides, music, as well as fighting or not fighting the disease.[16] It also chimes with the argument made by the anthropologist Mary Douglas in her book *How Institutions Think*.[17] She shows that life-and-death decisions in medical practice are made not by an individual calculating the merits of the particular case, but by following the path set out by the accepted values, vocabularies, and patterns of thinking in a social institution. The same logic applies to stopping pandemics.

The first act in the 'Pandemic X' story is the 1990s. This consisted in making the point that we are not prepared. The crucial year was the year when *Outbreak* was filmed: 1994. In the annals of global health policy, Lederberg's April 1994 meeting in Geneva is seminal. It is particularly remembered for something that doesn't appear in the meeting record, namely instigating legal reform.[18] The WHO is an international organization governed by its member states, which meet every year in the World Health Assembly (WHA). Among other things, they have authority over the regulations that set states' obligations to report infectious disease outbreaks and respond to them. These regulations also determine what governments are permitted to do: measures such as restricting travel or trade, imposing quarantine and isolation. They originated in the international sanitary regulations of the 19th century, were refashioned after World War II, and then updated as the International Health Regulations (IHR) in 1969.[19] David Fidler, the historian of disease and law, describes how they arose from Europe's inter-state order, which dates back to the 1648 Treaty of Westphalia, which established the rule whereby sovereign states didn't interfere in one another's domestic affairs:

> In keeping with the Westphalian template, the IHR constitute rules of international law created by states. The rules respect the principle of non-intervention by addressing only aspects of infectious diseases that relate to the intercourse among states. The IHR do not address aspects of public

health governance that touch on how a government prevents and controls infectious diseases in its sovereign territory.[20]

Both the principles and the list of 'notifiable diseases' had hardly changed since the first international sanitary conference in Paris in 1851. The IHR listed cholera, plague, and yellow fever. Smallpox had been removed from the list when it was eradicated. No new diseases had been added. The system was no longer fit for purpose.

The Lederberg meeting was held within the headquarters of the WHO, a modernist version of the classical architecture beloved of earlier medical institution-builders, in a city steeped in a culture of bureaucratic multilateralism. The WHO works by consensus, which means slowly. The IHR don't have the force of law: they are norms that rely on governments, jealous guardians of their own sovereign privileges, to act with goodwill and enlightened self-interest. States were obliged to report outbreaks of these diseases, which would require them to impose containment measures such as restrictions on travel and trade and allow other states to do the same. The list was outdated and too short. Relying on a definitive diagnosis of one of the notifiable diseases was a problem, because decisive action was needed early in an outbreak, and identifying the pathogen could take some time. Fast-moving contagions were coming to be seen as international security problems, and no country wanted its national security hostage to a foreign government that either didn't have the necessary medical capabilities or wanted to keep its sicknesses quiet. But the list was there, and if the WHO opened it up for renegotiation, the same problems that had recurred at every international health negotiation over the previous 150 years would reappear.

This cluster of problems was highlighted by plague in India just five months later. Among the fearsome qualities of plague is its habit of reappearing without warning. The plague disappeared from Europe in the 18th century and from the Central Asian republics of the Soviet Union in the mid-20th century. A hundred years ago, it was as big a killer in India as influenza or cholera and there were recurrent outbreaks until shortly after independence in 1947. After a 30-year absence, it unexpectedly returned in September 1994 when cases were diagnosed near the city of Surat.[21] What probably happened is the following. An earthquake caused villagers to temporarily abandon their grain stores, leaving rodents to feast undisturbed. Rats proliferated and in one place the plague bacillus multiplied with them. This was not a dangerous strain. In fact, had it occurred in any previous century it would hardly have registered at all: there were 6,500 cases and 56 people died. But when government medical officers announced that the disease was indeed plague, it caused panic. A quarter of the population of Surat abandoned the city. The state of Gujarat was cut off from the world. India itself faced a cascade of restrictions on travel and trade, with economic costs amounting to perhaps $2 billion. The chaos was compounded by a confused WHO response and a dispute over whether the disease was indeed plague or something else. The Surat outbreak came a few months too late for Laurie Garrett to include in her first book, *The Coming Plague*, so she opened her second book, *Betrayal of Trust*, with a chapter recounting this story. She concludes: 'In every possible way the essential public health trusts between authorities, science, medicine and the global populace were violated during the 1994 plague outbreak in India.'[22]

Plague was the quintessential *re-emerging* disease: an old scourge returning, as it were, from the grave. The Surat outbreak is a vivid example of how the fear unleashed by a pathogen can be more damaging than the microbe itself, which in this case luckily failed to live up to its virulent reputation. With a well-coordinated national and international response, beginning with simple antibiotic treatments, this outbreak could have passed with almost no illness or disruption. The problem, as Garrett insisted, was a breakdown of people's confidence in public health – a *justifiable* breakdown.

The Indian government did most things wrong, except that it immediately declared plague – an announcement that caused alarm and chaos.

If the Surat plague wasn't the Black Death, neither is contemporary African cholera the deadly cholera of the 19th century. It's a very nasty diarrhoeal disease that can be treated with oral hydration therapy. For example, the 2006 outbreak in Ethiopia had a case fatality rate of 1.1 per cent. According to official figures, it killed 44 people – probably an undercount, but not by much. The government led a public health response that contained the outbreak and treated patients.[23] Ethiopia called it 'acute watery diarrhoea' to avoid the stigma and the risk of having to shut down the country. This became standard practice in African countries, such as Zimbabwe (where the government response was less adequate and the fatality rate was higher).[24] Some other countries, such as Sierra Leone, did declare cholera because it helped bring in international aid.

The bigger problem with the IHR was new diseases that weren't on the list. The IHR could have been expanded on a disease-by-disease basis but this also posed problems. A technical difficulty was delay: if it took months for India to identify the very well-known plague bacterium, how long might it take for a puzzling new pathogen? The political issue was that the IHR were the property of the WHA and getting the Assembly to agree to new notifiable diseases was going to be even slower. Instead, the experts assembled in Geneva decided on a much more thorough overhaul, to create a new system of obligatory and immediate (24-hour) notification of outbreaks of known and unknown infectious agents.[25] They also proposed that the WHO should be allowed to receive reports from non-governmental sources, such as voluntary agencies and private physicians. China objected to this, and still does.

Internal WHO assessments following on from the Lederberg meeting were the basis for a resolution at the 1995 WHA, to revise and update the IHR. It took 10 years for the 194 WHA member states to adopt the new regulations, and it took the shock of SARS to make them act. The science was the easy part, the diplomacy was the difficult bit. Other things happened in the meantime. Energetic staff were assigned to the global surveillance system for outbreaks of infectious diseases, which hadn't been updated since the 1950s, and had languished as routine chores in Geneva and Atlanta. In 1997, the WHO's freshened-up report counted 60 'significant' outbreaks of both familiar and new diseases.[26] Virologists began talking about the 'Big One': the outbreak with the potential to go pandemic and kill millions.

That year there was an outbreak of avian influenza in Hong Kong. The strain – known as H5N1 – was extremely virulent in birds and there was reason to fear that it might be just as virulent in humans. The case fatality rate was high; fortunately the transmission rate was low. Eighteen people were infected and six died. The outbreak was contained.[27] In stark contrast to the shambles of the response to the Surat plague, Hong Kong showed the world that the system could work. Margaret Chan was Director of Health in Hong Kong at the time. After a brief hesitation in which she underplayed the first few cases, she ordered the cull of every chicken in the territory: 1.5 million in all. Chan was caught in the dilemma of pre-emption: being blamed for over-hyping a threat if it doesn't happen, and for underplaying it if it does. A dutiful civil servant with little public profile and no discernible political ambition, Chan was in a position that was even more delicate because of the contentious politics of Hong Kong at the time of handover from British colonial rule to China's uneasy 'one country, two systems' compromise. As the outbreak erupted, she was vilified in the media, but when it died away, she was praised. She was an accidental bureaucratic hero. This later won her elevation to head the WHO.

This was a moment in history in which dull bureaucracy was at its most prestigious – anything that tasted of order was palatable, as long as it wasn't the rot of anarchy. The Hong Kong outbreak was drained of political drama and turned into a lesson in the better functioning of public administration; the coordination of information systems among governments; enhanced contingency procedures for diagnosing pathogenic viruses in places with limited bio-security laboratory facilities; better-aligned emergency vaccine production regulations; and speeded-up supply chains for pharmaceutical products.[28] For the general public, this message was: the system is working, no need to worry and we can rely on science to solve our problem. It was the concluding part of Wald's 'outbreak narrative' with its reassuring ending. Chan didn't speak about 'war' on influenza. The leaders of a former colony integrated into an emerging superpower, with fragile protections on their freedoms, had a lifetime's schooling in avoiding martial language – that was the speciality of the Chinese Communist Party.

The official roadmap for pandemic preparedness planning was plotted out in the Hong Kong recommendations. The unofficial route map was: go directly to biomedicine and containment but don't go down any road that might disrupt the world's corporate production and trade system. Some biomedical lessons of Hong Kong flu were acted upon, others not. The biggest failure was vaccine research and production. The problem here is the non-existent commercial incentives for vaccine development for diseases that haven't infected people yet. Time and again, this elementary question of private companies providing public goods (or failing to do so) has arisen; time and again it has not been solved. Big pharma's profits are elsewhere.

The containment plans were focused on the virus, not the ecology that produced it. The premise of the influenza preparedness system is that these new strains of influenza will emerge, and there's nothing that can be done to stop them emerging – the tasks are to catch them quickly and stop them spreading. That's correct insofar as viral mutation is a fact of evolutionary life. But the fast pace at which new mutations are emerging, and the vastly increased risk that any one of them will become pandemic, isn't an irreducible fact of nature. Rather it's the result of how governments and corporations construct the artificial ecology of urbanization and industrial farming. One reason for the initial emergence and spread of the Hong Kong flu was genetic homogeneity of chickens, which provided an ecosystem for the accelerated evolution of flu viruses.[29] The slaughter of Hong Kong's chickens may have stopped the 1997 outbreak, but culling domestic poultry actually worsens this ecological incubator problem. Both family-owned backyard chickens and commercially farmed chickens are slaughtered. The small producers get their compensation too late to rebuild their businesses (if they get anything at all). The large commercial chicken farmers survive and even benefit: they are first in line for the bail-out money and they can move quickly to gobble up the vacant market share. For the world's biggest meat producers, the 1997 turmoil in the poultry market was an opportunity. They emerged bigger.[30] The corporate consolidation of poultry farming is a socio-economic problem. The conditions under which those birds are farmed is an ecological and public health calamity in waiting.

This is an example of how systems are designed to manage identified and measured risks, even if that means allowing unmeasured dangers to increase. A similar problem arises in economists' pandemic preparedness. Peter Sands, whose career switched from the head of a bank and having a personal interest in public health, to being head of the Global Fund to Fight AIDS, Tuberculosis, and Malaria, has explained how difficult it is for public health experts and economists to speak to one another.[31] He observes that there are well-known cognitive biases at work when we try to assess a low-probability, high-impact event (shark attacks, terrorist crimes, earthquakes). A deeper problem is that economists can only deal with the kinds of quantifiable risks that fit their models, particularly equilibrium models. They simply can't hear what pandemic preparedness people are telling them. It's an irony our everyday vocabulary and grammar struggle to deal with. What a historian of epidemics calls a 'certainty' is excluded from economic forecasts as a 'radical uncertainty' – even though there are enough outbreaks, epidemics, and pandemics for any student of economic history to gnaw away at. The two ways of analysing the world seem to be incommensurable. Such is the power of economic models – the deep socialization of the norm of economistic thinking – that their way of seeing the world persisted throughout every crisis until Covid-19.

Pandemic Preparedness Meets Bio-Terror

In the 1990s, western security analysts were more amenable to creative rethinking, following the disappearance of their strategic adversary. After the end of the Cold War, the US national security establishment contemplated emerging and re-emerging threats, including failing states, terrorist groups, transnational organized crime, nuclear proliferation, the Y2K bug, emerging great power rivalry, and infectious diseases. International public health people were promoting the 'security threat' framework to get more political attention. The military and security people gave it a half-hearted embrace, as they didn't consider disease a proper security threat. Reports from the National Intelligence Council and CIA had raised the profile of pandemic threats, but not to the top tier.

The security establishment had developed a way of thinking about extreme singular events and making politicians listen. They did it through a collaborative storytelling method. This was crucial, not only because it put pandemics in among the high-priority threats, but also because the under-examined assumptions in the script came to define pandemic response. Four institutions in the orbit of the security establishment, convened by the Johns Hopkins Center for Biodefense, planned a vivid exercise to highlight the threat. They called it 'Operation Dark Winter' and it was an adaptation of the war-gaming simulations pioneered by the RAND corporation in the 1960s to explore how political leaders would respond under the stresses of a nuclear war. Dark Winter simulated a bioterrorist attack using weaponized smallpox.[32] The designers drew on epidemiological data for a smallpox epidemic to construct a plausible scenario. They used simulated news broadcasts, plotted out secondary crises sparked by bewildered state governors and panicked crowds, and brought in real (retired) decision-makers to play key roles. Former Senator Sam Nunn played the president; James Woolsey reprised his position as CIA director. There were a hundred observers. Using actual information for vaccine stocks, hospital capacities, and the logistical capabilities of the national guard and other emergency response agencies, the scenario unfolded into an out-of-control national epidemic that caused social and political chaos. It ended darkly with no conclusion save a question mark.

Dark Winter was held over three days in June 2001. Its frightening unfinished scenario became a legend among those who participated. The next challenge was: how to energize politicians and the public to prepare for a threat that is devastating but hypothetical? One that can be foreseen by experts but is beyond the horizon of our everyday imaginings? Scientists may have learned to read data and risk, including those risks that can't really be quantified, and assemble them into narratives that make sense to them. But it is notoriously difficult to motivate people to think clearly about improbable calamities. What's needed is a leader who can muse, 'Reports that say that something hasn't happened are always interesting to me.' Donald Rumsfeld said those words a few moments before his much-better known rumination, on 'known knowns', 'known unknowns', and 'unknown unknowns – the ones we don't know we don't know'.[33] Rumsfeld was talking about Iraq's alleged weapons of mass destruction, but the thinking extended to other threats, including microbes. Poetry, philosophy – it was also pandemic preparedness. Except that it would be more accurate to describe Pathogen X as an *imagined* unknown.

No fictionalized dramatization is needed here. In the annals of anti-state terrorism, this was the Big One. The crimes committed by Al-Qaeda on 11 September 2001 put America's, and the world's, security agenda on a new track. This included not just conventional military action and espionage, but also the global health and security agenda. In the words of Tom Bossert, who worked for President George W. Bush in the White House: 'There was a realization that it's no longer fantastical to raise scenarios about planes falling from the sky, or anthrax arriving in the mail. . . . It was not a novel. It was the world we were living.'[34] The Bush administration wanted to know the worst, wanted to prepare for every calamity, however improbable, especially if it could be weaponized by terrorists. This was a moment when '1 per cent' threats could be a priority agenda.

The anthrax scare in the weeks following 9/11 made it real. Letters containing spores of the disease were sent to politicians in Washington, DC. Five people died, 17 others fell sick. Anthrax wasn't 'Disease X': it was a known pathogen and a favoured bio-warfare agent. But it was, at minimum, 'Outbreak X': a dangerous bacterium unexpectedly spread by a new vector, in this case the US Postal Service. The anthrax outbreak was a detective story for real: who sent the contaminated letters and why? The FBI assembled the 'Amerithrax' task force of 25 full-time investigators who worked for seven years. But the case was never properly resolved, because the suspect, a mentally disturbed rogue scientist called Bruce Ivins, committed suicide in 2008 before he was apprehended. The FBI report makes clear that Ivins was the sole suspect and that they believed that he acted alone.[35] As with other prominent 'sole gunman' cases, there has been conspiracy theorizing about the anthrax case, but the case against Ivins is strong. His motive was never clear. It seems plausible that he wanted to make the point that bio-terror was a real and neglected danger, and if that was indeed his plan, he succeeded.

The seeds of bio-fear had been sown on well-prepared

soil: Operation Dark Winter looked prescient. The White House demanded urgent measures against bio-terrorism and provided a $6 billion annual budget for preventing outbreaks of weaponized germs, including smallpox and anthrax. Every infectious disease specialist knew that a naturally occurring epidemic and a bio-terror outbreak would have the same effects and need the same response – and that a natural outbreak was much more probable. When the CDC was allocated its (relatively small) share of the money, it 'put the vast majority into bolstering an underfunded public-health infrastructure. The rationale was that the nation had little chance of fighting a bioterror attack without a strong system for detecting, reporting and treating any emerging infectious disease.'[36] This rationale was absorbed into national security thinking and stayed there for the Obama administration as well. The section on countering biological threats in the 2010 National Security Strategy recognized 'Pandemics and Infectious Disease' as security threats, but its proposals kept national global public health programmes with public health specialists, mostly civilian.[37]

The aftermath of 9/11 was a rare occasion on which political leaders could take institutional action, spend money, and also shape public thinking about an as-yet-unrealized threat. The institutions, funds, and rhetoric were all shaped to fit the 'war on terror' – to be specific, the ways in which the Bush administration reoriented America towards a pervasive and permanent counter-terror mobilization. Initially, fear of militant jihadists subsumed everything, and the Federal Emergency Management Agency was placed under the Department of Homeland Security, leaving it ill prepared for Hurricane Katrina in August 2005. The possibility of a huge storm making landfall on a major city had long been foreseen, but preparedness had been neglected. When it happened, it was a reminder and an analogy for other possible disasters.[38] President Bush, speaking at the National Institutes of Health in November 2005, warned that pandemic influenza was potentially the biggest such threat facing America. Bush compared an outbreak to a forest fire and then went on to use other words that resonated with him and his audience:

> Our country has been given fair warning of this danger to our homeland – and time to prepare. . . . By preparing now, we can give our citizens some peace of mind knowing that our nation is ready to act at the first sign of danger, and that we have the plans in place to prevent and, if necessary, withstand an influenza pandemic.[39]

Viruses Are Things of Beauty

When virologists became drawn into the world of biosecurity, we needed to be concerned, not just because they're dealing with extremely dangerous pathogens but also because of how some of them may see the human world. The cognitive and institutional structure of biosecurity gave them great latitude to explore and experiment. In *The Hot Zone*, Preston imaginatively reconstructs the thoughts of virologist Tom Geisbert as he contemplated the first images of the Reston Ebola virus.

> He saw virus particles shaped like snakes, in negative images. They were white cobras tangled among themselves, like the hair of Medusa. They were the face of Nature herself, the obscene goddess revealed naked. This life form thing was breathtakingly beautiful. As he stared at it, he found himself being pulled out of the human world into a world where moral boundaries blur and finally dissolve completely. He was lost in wonder and admiration, even though he knew that he was the prey.[40]

In this book, I have made some simple forays into seeing the world from a microbe's point of view, anthropomorphizing pathogens so as to help us consider the logic of radically different perspectives on reality. This can be a useful mental prosthesis. But the more precise the model, the more strongly the conclusion depends on the assumptions, stated and unstated. Preston also recalls his own conversation with Karl Johnson, who headed the international mission to Zaïre in 1976 and whom he joined fly fishing in Montana.

> [Preston]: 'Are you worried about a species-threatening event?'
> [Johnson] stared at me, 'What the hell do you mean by that?'
> 'I mean a virus that wipes us out.'

Preston observes that a virus can be useful to a species by 'thinning it out'. He continues his exchange with Johnson, asking:

> 'Do you find viruses beautiful?'
> 'Oh yeah,' he said softly. 'Isn't it true that if you stare into the eyes of a cobra, the fear has another side to it? The fear is lessened as you begin to see the essence of the beauty.'[41]

Those who study a topic in great depth come to understand it in a way that others do not. With deep insight comes a kind of rewiring of cognition, a fine-tuning of intuition, that mimics the logic of the subject itself.

Let me take the parallel of the atomic bomb. The Manhattan Project, which developed the first atom bomb in the spring of 1945, was a scientific venture into the unknown. For those involved, it was thrilling: exciting and terrifying. The scientists in the desert had the trust and backing of the US president and were working on the biggest intellectual and practical challenge of their lifetimes at a moment in history in which civilization was in the balance. The physicists were exploring the limits of existence and the boundaries of annihilation. Watching the Trinity test, Robert Oppenheimer said, 'Now I am become death, the destroyer of worlds.' The day before, his colleague Enrico Fermi, nicknamed 'the Pope' for the purported infallibility of his calculations, 'took wagers from his fellow scientists on the question of whether the first atomic bomb test would ignite the atmosphere, and if so, whether it would merely destroy New Mexico or destroy the world'.[42] Oppenheimer, Fermi, and their colleagues were taking risks that only they could formulate and which they certainly weren't allowed to communicate beyond themselves. They were like mountaineers scaling uncharted peaks, exhilarated by both the danger and the triumph, ultimately coming to a point at which they sought out new summits simply because they were there to be climbed. Another physicist on the project, Edward Teller, later became obsessed with constructing bigger and bigger bombs, because he could.

This intellectual culture, combined with the secrecy and defensiveness of the military command responsible for nuclear weapons, didn't change at the end of World War II; it didn't change throughout the Cold War; and it hasn't gone away. Fermi's 1945 wager was won: the test didn't destroy either New Mexico or the world, and there hasn't been a nuclear war, deliberate or inadvertent, since August 1945. But physicists are profoundly aware of the original sin of unlocking the secrets of the universe. 'Normal accident theory'[43] predicts that, sooner or later, a devastating accident will happen involving a nuclear weapon. And there is a list of accidents and near misses, caused by mixtures of human error and technical malfunction, that make for truly terrifying reading. Eric Schlosser, who compiled a minute-by-minute account of the accident involving a Titan II nuclear missile at Damascus, Arkansas, in September 1980, describes how it was set in motion by a trivial event (a technician dropping a tool during routine maintenance, which struck a missile's fuel tank at a crucially bad angle, causing a leak), compounded by the way in which a tightly coupled and interactive system rapidly meant that the danger escalated (the leaked fuel in the enclosed rocket chamber was likely to ignite as the temperature rose), and the lack of clear on-the-spot information and an inflexible response system.

None of these were singularly to blame (especially not the 21-year-old whose grip on his wrench slipped). Schlosser concludes that, by good fortune, 'none of those leaks and accidents led to a nuclear disaster. But if one had, the disaster wouldn't have been inexplicable or hard to comprehend. It would have made perfect sense.'[44]

Biological weapons systems are candidates for 'normal accidents' like this. So too advanced virological research, which has the special twist that its highest-altitude climbers are driven not only by intellectual thrill but also by the noble motive of mastering the deadliest diseases. They are a small group who know each other well and are fiercely self-protective. Virologists don't like to fully admit dangers in their research, from the collection and transport of samples, to laboratory work and storage. Perhaps we shouldn't be surprised that we have to turn to the journal set up in 1945 for public discussion of the dangers of 'the Pandora's Box of modern science',[45] the *Bulletin of the Atomic Scientists*, to find the most candid discussion on this topic. Bio-weapons specialist Martin Furmanski writes, 'Many laboratory escapes of high-consequence pathogens have occurred, resulting in transmission beyond laboratory personnel. Ironically, these laboratories were working with pathogens to prevent the very outbreaks they ultimately caused. For that reason, the tragic consequences have been called "self-fulfilling prophecies."'[46] There is one case, not well known but generally accepted among virologists, of a laboratory virus going pandemic. This happened in 1977 when a strain of H1N1 influenza virus suddenly reappeared after a 25-year absence. When genetic analysis later became possible, scientists realized something very unusual about this re-emergent influenza: '[I]t was genetically similar, though not identical, to an H1N1 isolate from 1950. Initially it was suggested that this virus could have lain dormant or evolved slowly in non-human hosts for decades, but it is now generally assumed that the virus was kept frozen in a yet unidentified laboratory.'[47] This is an understatement: in the wild, it would have evolved, and given that the rate of influenza's evolutionary mutation is about one million times faster than that of human beings, it is as though a mammalian ancestor from 25 million years ago had unexpectedly appeared, an event with a natural probability approaching vanishing point. The laboratory has never been traced and the circumstances of the release aren't known: was it a vaccine trial that went wrong, or a laboratory accident? It was probably in Russia or China, and some have consoled themselves that this was the era before the most rigorous biosafety protocols were introduced.[48]

There have been other cases, including smallpox (in Birmingham in 1978) Venezuelan equine encephalitis in 1995, SARS outbreaks after the SARS epidemic (twice), and Foot and Mouth disease in the UK. Most of these cases occurred through human error.[49] The 2001 anthrax outbreak could also be considered a 'normal accident', although it was deliberate – not every person authorized to have access to lethal pathogens will be mentally stable.

The greatest dangers may occur with the research that aims to produce a vaccine. The main reason is that for obvious reasons vaccine research focuses on deadly pathogens, both familiar viruses and likely candidates for pandemic potential. If the researcher's goal is to identify Pathogen X before it goes pandemic, then that pathogen has to be tracked down in its naturally existing state and examined in a laboratory. That's already a hazard. Given that the biggest danger is that an existing pathogen mutates to become transmissible to humans, transmissible among humans, and more virulent, the virus hunters have to disassemble the viruses they have collected and explore how they could naturally reassemble to gain these deadly characteristics. That's an even greater hazard.

The dangers are further increased when artificially enhanced viruses are involved. This was especially salient with 'gain of function' experiments, which manipulate viruses in the laboratory to see whether and how they can become more transmissible or more virulent. The logic is that if we can identify the most crucial elements in a virus, for example those that allow it to infect human cells, then we can develop a vaccine more effectively. This became controversial when researchers experimented with H5N1 in 2011, and the journal *Science* hesitated before agreeing to publish their paper. What the reviewers were concerned about was not the quality of the science, but the ethics. The University of Wisconsin-Madison news release explained:

> 'Our study shows that relatively few amino acid mutations are sufficient for a virus with an avian H5 hemagglutinin to acquire the ability to transmit in mammals,' says Yoshihiro Kawaoka, a University of Wisconsin-Madison flu researcher whose study of H5N1 virus transmissibility was at the center of the debate. 'This study has significant public health benefits and contributes to our understanding of this important pathogen. By identifying mutations that facilitate transmission among mammals, those whose job it is to monitor viruses circulating in nature can look for these mutations so measures can be taken to effectively protect human health.'[50]

Critics argued that engineering these dangerous traits into a virus was reckless – at the very least, there needed to be a fuller debate on the topic.[51] Even publishing the blueprint for a more lethal virus could be a form of release, because it would allow a malign researcher to reproduce the experiment.[52] The US National Institutes of Health ordered a suspension of this line of research while it convened an expert group to investigate. The National Science Advisory Board for Biosecurity commissioned a detailed assessment of risks and benefits, convened two symposia, wrote new ethics guidelines, and published a thousand-page report. This tried to balance pandemic preparedness research against biosafety. The outcome was, as Andrew Lakoff writes, that 'the catastrophic scenario at the heart of the former outstripped the regulatory capacities of the latter.'[53] The report came out in June 2016, and six months later the moratorium on gain of function research was lifted.[54] Research virologists lament that they lost two years of research time, and at least one has made the case that this disastrously slowed research into coronaviruses in bats.[55]

The perils of virological research aren't just within the laboratory. Virus hunters take risks – some of them as simple as not isolating themselves when they show symptoms of fever when working with dangerous microbes.[56] David Quammen has described bat-capture expeditions into caves in China and Uganda which are frankly terrifying, not only because of the risks of zoonotic infection through a bat bite or scratch, or just touching bat faeces, but also because of poisonous snakes and rockfalls.[57] Virus hunters are brave; they do it for the intellectual excitement, the moral commitment, the professional prestige, and the thrill of the chase. Some are also extraordinarily, perhaps naïvely, hopeful. Peter Daszak, whose organization EcoHealth Alliance is a world leader in the field, has said: 'I'm optimistic about this. I think that in 50 years we will look back on this age and say, we were in the pandemic era but we dealt with it.'[58] Such a sunny mindset might lead a researcher to think that short-term risks are worth taking.

Another way of formulating the question of risk is to ask: what is being protected by the risk-taking? I suggest that the ecology of the Anthropocene and the social and economic organization of our human population are intrinsically pathogenic, and that in order to preserve this dangerous structure, we encourage highly targeted risk-taking by those who we hope will protect us from the most immediate dangers. We are creating enemies and then manufacturing dangerous weapons to fight them. In the first two decades of this century, several pathogens passed the first screening as candidates for Pandemic X, but none of them quite fitted. The rest of this chapter examines three. After HIV, SARS was the first truly emerging pathogen, and in retrospect the 2003 outbreak was a test run for Covid-19 in both virology and politics. Avian influenza and swine flu thankfully didn't realize their widely feared potential. Ebola did go epidemic but was handled, not as an international health security crisis but as a challenge for biomedical humanitarianism.

SARS: Storylines for Outbreak X

With the hindsight of 2020, it is tempting to write the story of every recent outbreak of a new infectious pathogen as the precursor pandemic-that-nearly-was. In the case of SARS – severe acute respiratory syndrome – in 2002–3, that would be fair, because the virology and politics of the outbreak have obvious similarities to Covid-19, and because the story was written that way at the time. In their introduction to their short book *SARS: Prelude to Pandemic*, Arthur Kleinman and James Watson wrote: 'In retrospect, SARS is probably best seen as a harbinger of future events that might be catastrophic for the global system as we know it today. . . . This book thus has a didactic agenda with the broadest possible policy implications: Can we avoid the Big One?'[59]

The virus now known as SARS-CoV-1 was the first virulent coronavirus known to science; it jumped the species barrier from its natural host (bats), possibly through an intermediate mammalian host (pangolins); it is a respiratory infection that can spread quickly; the speed of contagion was faster than the scientific development of therapy and vaccine; it broke out in southern China and the authorities delayed in alerting the world for several critical months; it travelled overland from mainland China to Hong Kong and from there by aeroplane to Singapore and Canada; and the containment response involved shutting down air travel and imposing quarantine on entire cities. It's different from its cousin SARS-CoV-2 (which causes Covid-19) in two major ways. It's a more lethal disease, killing about 15 per cent of those it infects. However, crucial to its containment, patients become infectious only when their symptoms begin. This feature makes it much easier to identify those who are capable of transmitting the disease to others and thereby contain the outbreaks.

Reality came first, then the movie: *Contagion* (directed by Steven Soderbergh and released in 2011). The fictional viral protagonist is called MEV-1, is more readily transmissible than SARS, and has a higher fatality rate (25 per cent). *Contagion* is the most thoroughly researched epidemic movie ever made and the science is plausible, thus making it, along with *Outbreak*, a notable exception among cinematic representations of infectious disease outbreaks.

How the SARS epidemic was contained is a story of three interlocking institutions, each of which thought and acted in different ways: China, the WHO, and the US national security apparatus. In November 2002, doctors in Foshan city, Guangdong province, began noticing what they called 'atypical pneumonia'. As a new disease, there was no established procedure for classifying and reporting it according to the protocols of China's Law on Prevention and Treatment of Infectious Diseases.[60] According to the Implementing Regulations on the State Secrets Law, 'any occurrence of infectious diseases should be classified as a state secret' before it is 'announced by the Ministry of Health or organs authorized by the Ministry'. In other words, until such time as the Ministry chose to make information about the disease public, any physician or journalist who reported on the disease would risk being prosecuted for leaking state secrets.[61] The public health system had abandoned the Mao-era emphasis on equitable primary health care for all in favour of a more individualistic and curative approach, but hadn't moved away from an ethos of treating information as a privilege to be carefully husbanded by the vanguard party.

The cover-up was less a centrally orchestrated concealment and more the normal operation of a complex bureaucracy in which there was every incentive not to pass on bad news. In February 2003, the authorities admitted that there was an outbreak of a new disease but concealed the numbers, especially those infected in Beijing. By this time, infectious disease specialists at the WHO and CDC suspected that something untoward was happening. Within China, most crucial was the disgust among a handful of Chinese doctors who began leaking the information that hundreds of patients were being admitted to hospital with this new disease. The information shutdown was particularly tight during the preparations for the National People's Congress, which opened on 3 March. This was a huge political event, a transition in power that happened once every 10 years, and the media diligently suppressed all bad news. On 19 March, President Hu Jintao and Premier Wen Jiabao were sworn into office. These new leaders turned the epidemic crisis into a tactical opportunity. The crisis was both the disease itself and the fast-developing political fiasco caused by messages circulating on the internet. The Communist Party tradition was to suppress dissent, admit no mistakes, and ride out the crisis. This time it was more difficult because the disease had already spread beyond China's borders, reaching Hong Kong, Singapore, and Canada, and the WHO had been alerted.

The Director General at the time was Gro Harlem Brundtland. A former prime minister of Norway, she was well aware of the limits of her authority as head of an intergovernmental organization whose member states carefully guarded their governments' rights to take emergency action. She knew the political risks run by a UN agency head who overstepped the mark. But she also knew what was at stake and was ready to grasp a solution beyond the reach of law. The new international health regulations were still in draft form, becalmed in committee. However, the rationale for them, including taking information from non-governmental sources, immediate notification of new diseases, and WHO leadership in alerting the world, had already been discussed at seven successive meetings of the WHA and innumerable other conferences. The norms were running ahead of the law – and the virus was running even faster. On 12 March, the

WHO issued an alert about 'atypical pneumonia' in China and asked to send a team to investigate. China agreed. Three days later, the WHO named the new disease 'SARS'. Then on 2 April, in an astonishing rebuke to Beijing, without precedent, Brundtland issued the WHO's first ever travel advisory for China.[62] This not only threatened the Chinese economy but also embarrassed the Chinese leadership.[63] One reason for Brundtland's fearlessness was that she was in her final months as Director General; her successor, who was the Chinese public health expert Dr Lee Jong-wook, would have found it much harder to criticize Beijing.

Shortly afterwards, Brundtland also issued a travel advisory for Toronto, in effect warning the Canadian government to shut down its largest city. Jean Chrétien, a Liberal prime minister with an international outlook, was ready to comply. It worked. China and Hong Kong had recent experience in military-style lockdowns and China was a police state in any case; Singapore was run on similar lines. But no western city had ever experienced this kind of *de facto* martial rule since World War II.

David Fidler calls SARS the 'first post-Westphalian pathogen'.[64] Sara Davies and colleagues see this as the tipping point in the cascade of the updated IHR's new norms – the socialization of fresh thinking about global public health. Brundtland was careful to frame the disease as a security threat needing a cooperative response of sovereign states.[65] But the context of the war on terror and the concurrent US invasion of Iraq were crucial too. The post-9/11 investments in surveillance systems and rapid response to biological threats meant that the United States was already on alert, so that emerging infectious diseases couldn't be kept secret, and even a country as powerful as China was keen not to offend Washington.[66]

SARS was also an opportunity for Hu Jintao and the new leadership to impose their authority in a distinctive way. They debated the issue intensely. The *Washington Post* summarized what happened next:

On April 17, Hu took the plunge. During an unscheduled meeting of the all-powerful Politburo of the Communist Party, he acknowledged the government had lied about the disease and committed the Communist Party to an all-out war against an epidemic sweeping the capital and the country. Three days later, China's Communist leadership carried out its most significant political purge since the crackdown around Tiananmen Square in 1989. The capital's mayor and the country's health minister were fired for covering up the epidemic. [67]

Campaign rhetoric is what the Chinese Communist Party does in times of crisis. The government declared 'war on SARS'[68] and was mocked by citizens using social media and samizdat, including through subversive parodies of Mao's poetic style.[69]

Worldwide, about 8,100 people are known to have been infected with SARS and 774 died. Chinese official numbers – underestimates for sure – record that it infected more than 5,300 people and killed 349. The lockdowns and other disruptions cost the world about $40 billion in economic losses.[70] The consensus is that the containment measures were slow to get started but worked. China's response was mostly low-tech isolation measures enforced by a pyramid of people's committees with disciplinary powers, with some new electronic surveillance methods tried out as well.[71] Most of those who wrote the story of SARS were interested in epidemic diseases, and their verdict was that it showed the potential for a new global public health security order.[72] Political scientists were more cautious. Shortly after the epidemic, Tony Saich asked whether SARS was 'China's Chernobyl or much ado about nothing?'[73] At that time, he reserved judgement, concluding that the Chinese authorities *ought* to learn.

Seventeen years on, Saich's assessment of the response to Covid-19 was, '[N]o, they didn't learn from the SARS epidemic.'[74] That is a public health verdict. The lessons that the Chinese government learned were *political* ones. To them, the biggest cost of SARS was reputational. It was just as important to control the narrative as to control the virus. So, while the government invested in technical surveillance of emerging viruses and scientific research, it didn't lighten the apparatus for censorship and it began reeling the WHO back into the Westphalian net. The medical anthropologist Christos Lynteris recounts a conversation he had with a Chinese epidemiologist – a medical professor and an officer in a government disease control department. Lynteris asked him whether SARS might make a comeback. 'We do not really know, he replied, why it went or where it's gone. But what will you do if SARS returns one day? I retorted. In a tone perched between a lament and a scoff, the epidemiologist replied: *Exactly what we did last time*.'[75]

Influenza: How to Name a Pandemic?

'Severe acute respiratory syndrome' was named by committee in Geneva in March 2003. It was chosen in part because that was what physicians had called it, and partly so as not to offend China, and thereby help gain Chinese cooperation. This marked a new era for naming pathogens: until then, like Victorian-era adventurers, microbiologists could choose their own names. When cases of Ebola broke out in the southern Sudanese town of Maridi, '[I]t was first called Maridi disease, then haemorrhagic febrile disease, Green Monkey disease, and finally Marburg.'[76] (It later turned out that Marburg and Ebola viruses are distinct.) Peter Piot describes how the international team dispatched to Zaïre in 1976 hit on the name 'Ebola':

> Late one night we were drinking Karl [Johnson]'s Kentucky bourbon – it was one of those half-gallon bottles with a handle – discussing what our new virus should be named. Pierre [Sureau] argued for Yambuku virus, which had the advantage of simplicity; it was what most of us were already

calling the disease. But Joel [Breman] reminded us that naming killer diseases after specific places can be very stig-matizing; with Lassa virus, discovered in 1969 in a Nigerian town of that name, it had caused no end of problems to the people from that locality. Karl liked to call his viruses after rivers: he felt that took some of the sting out of the geo-graphical finger-pointing. It was what he had done when he'd discovered Machupo virus in Bolivia in 1959, and it was clear that night that he had every intention of doing the same in Zaïre.

But we couldn't call our virus after the majestic Congo River: a Congo-Crim virus already existed. Were there any other rivers near Yambuku? We charged en masse to a not-very-large map of Zaïre that was pinned up in the corridor. At that scale it looked as though the closest river to Yambuku was called Ebola – 'Black River' in Lingala. It seemed suitably ominous.

Actually there's no connection between the hemorrhagic fever and the Ebola River. Indeed, the Ebola River isn't even the closest river to the Yambuku mission. But in our entirely fatigued state, that's what we ended up calling the virus: Ebola.[77]

But for the presence of a woman in the group, the scene could have taken place a century earlier: a crowd of white people, drinking, clustered around a very large-scale map, choosing a name for a natural object.

No one is offended by the well-worn word 'influenza' or its expert H-N- typology, but influenza generated two revealing controversies over naming: 'swine flu' and 'pan-demic influenza'. In the first decade of the 2000s, influenza experts became more and more worried about the danger that a new subtype H5N1 strain of avian flu – culprit for the Hong Kong outbreak in 1997 – would be devastating not only in chickens but also in people. There was a slew of virological research papers and pandemic preparedness plans, and a book by Mike Davis, *The Monster at Our Door*, each of which predicted a high likelihood of a devastating pandemic. It was those danger signs flashing that were in the background of President Bush's November 2005 speech. It didn't happen. As before, H5N1 wasn't readily transmissible between people. Those who had sounded the warnings concluded that *Homo sapiens* had got lucky in the influenza reassortment lottery, that we had dodged a bullet.

Four years later came a new subtype of H1N1, a direct descendant of the 1918 virus, which had mutated in a pig in the Mexican village of LaGloria. Keeping huge numbers of pigs in close proximity in farms and feedlots provided plenty of opportunities for viral evolution in mammals, and H1N1 subtypes had been circulating among pigs ever since 1918. The WHO therefore adopted the name 'swine flu',[78] which avoided stigmatizing Mexico but caused another problem. Pig farmers complained about the name, because their business suffered as consumers assumed, mistakenly, that the virus could be transmitted by eating pork, rather than having emerged as a byproduct of their production methods. Many countries banned American pork and the United States lost 10 per cent of its pork export markets, worth about $13.6 million per week. The meat industry lobbied Congress. Senator Tom Harkin, Democrat of the farm state Iowa, convened a hearing on what he called 'the so-called swine flu', while pork producers launched a campaign to rename it 'North American influenza'.[79] The *New York Times* reported C. Larry Pope, the chief executive of Smithfield Foods, as saying: 'Swine flu is a misnomer. . . . They need to be concerned about influenza, but not eating pork.'[80] Two days after the hearings, the *National Hog Farmer* website was first with the news:

> The new hybrid flu strain affecting a number of countries will now be called '2009 H1N1 Flu,' according to the American Meat Institute (AMI). The decision to change the name of the virus – formerly known as swine flu – was announced by Health and Human Services Secretary Kathleen Sibelius,

Centers for Disease Control and Prevention acting chief Richard Besser and was repeated by others during a news briefing this morning.[81]

It wasn't the villagers living along the Ebola river in Congo, nor the people of the Zika forest in Uganda or the Nigerian town of Lassa, nor even the authorities in Hong Kong, who instigated this change, but American pig farmers. A few years later, the WHO decided, by consensus, to avoid using place names and animal names.[82] This was an extension of standard UN practice whereby the acronym for anything – a new agency, a new peacekeeping mission, or even a new office building – has to be run through a multi-lingual dictionary to make sure it won't have an offensive meaning in any known language. There were some critics, who said that names such as SARS and 2009 H1N1 weren't memorable and could be confusing, and that there were advantages to names such as 'Monkeypox' because they alerted people to the source of infection.[83] No one in the WHO committee needed to mention that had they had chosen the name 'Foshan virus' for SARS, it might not have helped gain China's cooperation. Following the guidelines, Middle East respiratory syndrome (MERS) wasn't 'camel virus' and SARS-CoV-2 isn't 'Wuhan virus'.

The new H1N1 strain of influenza prompted another and more theoretically challenging question: *what is a pandemic*? Today's everyday use of 'pandemic' is that it is a transcontinental epidemic with a terrible human impact. Until 2009, the WHO definition fitted this: 'An influenza pandemic occurs when a new influenza virus appears against which the human population has no immunity, resulting in several simultaneous epidemics worldwide with enormous numbers of deaths and illness.' But this definition faced the problem that the whole point of pandemic preparedness is to *prevent* a new virus from having this effect.[84] Instead, influenza specialists made the call on the basis of the novelty of the strain of the virus, rather than waiting for a threshold of fatalities to be crossed. According to this method, a mild variant would be defined as 'pandemic' if it were new and transmissible, which is exactly what happened with the new H1N1. It went pandemic and the CDC estimates that it killed between 151,700 and 575,400 people worldwide, about the same number as normal seasonal flu, albeit with a different (younger) age profile.[85] After being called out by a CNN reporter, the WHO quietly changed the definition on its website, dropping the 'enormous number of deaths and illness'.[86]

The WHO and governments that had spent billions preparing for pandemic influenza were blamed for wasting money and needlessly scaring people. One accusation was that they deliberately inflated the threat so as to boost pharmaceutical company profits. That wasn't true. Public health experts replied that it was better to have a response without a pandemic than a pandemic without a response. A more insightful critique was that the ecological conditions for viral evolution in the early 21st century weren't those of World War I and neither the 2005 H5 variant nor 2009 H1N1 had gone through comparable processes of natural selection for virulence and transmissibility among human hosts.[87] To which there were two counter-arguments. First, could not industrial pig and poultry farms and densely packed shanty towns, so common in many countries, also be incubators of monstrous new strains?[88] And second, of course, low risk doesn't mean zero risk, and any such danger will stay unlikely until it actually happens.

Political leaders had moved pandemic response into the political realm and were now struggling with a foreseeable outcome for which they had not prepared, namely managing the public relations fallout from pandemics-that-weren't. 'Disease X' was an everyday controversy in political business as usual. Why spend resources and generate anxieties without discernible political benefit? No politicians were served by the claim that they had invisibly saved lives. Poor countries wanted greater equity in dealing with actually existing health problems rather than catering to fears of the global north, especially if the new vaccines provided in response went first to richer countries. Indonesia refused to comply with its IHR obligations on the argument that there was no guarantee that if it identified a new strain of influenza, it would be at the front of the queue for a vaccine against that strain. Other developing countries were also unhappy that too much of the WHO agenda seemed to be set by a US-led concern with health security. They wanted the organization to focus on strengthening health systems and integrating health into development, rebalancing global health spending away from vertical programmes focused on specific diseases towards investing in health for all. This was a socially progressive set of tasks that included reducing inequalities in access to health, more collaborative ways of setting health policies, and increasing the role of communities in health provision. Under the leadership of Margaret Chan from 2006, the WHO didn't become any less political – but its politics changed. It embraced the politics of health-as-equitable-development and 'almost entirely willingly jettisoned its utilization of the health-as-security discourse'.[89]

The WHO didn't abandon pandemic preparedness, but its headquarters expected member states to take the lead in this politically risky area. In practice, this meant the United States first, followed by Europe and China. Health-as-security didn't go away, it just became more American. The CDC and other US government initiatives, such as USAID's Emerging Pandemic Threats Program, took on a greater burden of responsibility for leading the response to any dangerous outbreak. And while the WHO's broader health philosophy was admirably equitable and inclusive, it didn't extend those principles to pandemic prevention and preparedness. Many health professionals didn't like the new American 'war on disease' model, but rather than reforming it they decided to put their energies elsewhere.

The treatment of emerging pathogens as a security threat reflected some of the same weaknesses as President Bush's 'global war on terror'. The model was eternal vigilance for that rogue individual that can inflict catastrophic damage, which requires maintaining pervasive, intrusive, and worldwide intelligence and security institutions. It needed everyone to conform to a model designed by the world's richest countries to protect their own health and way of life. It required citizens and taxpayers in those rich countries to entrust governments with resources and powers that didn't bring immediate visible return. And perhaps most importantly, the model put an immense responsibility on infectious disease surveillance that it could not fulfil. Microbe hunters can only isolate a miniscule fraction of the pathogens with zoonotic potential. There are hundreds of infectious disease outbreaks every year, many of which involve patients with borderline 'atypical' symptoms. Putting the focus on the individual pathogen that emerges randomly from the viral mutation lottery with the wrong configuration is to accept an increasingly pathogenic terrain as a fact of life. In the same way that the 'war on terror' led to a futile effort to end the threat to America by killing supposed terrorists one by one while neglecting the socio-political milieu that produced them, so too the new 'war on disease' isolated the microbe and ignored the terrain. The model accepted that ecological-evolutionary factors, such as the dangers associated with urbanization, deforestation, or industrial farming, just meant that the dice in the mutational lottery were loaded. The model's premise was that the ecological privileges of contemporary metropolitan life – including air travel; global trade in foodstuffs and other natural products; offices and hotels with centralized ventilation systems; public gathering and mixing in markets, theatres, and mass transit systems – were non-negotiable. We would adjust to the pandemic only when it actually arrived. Was this the right approach? These were public conversations we didn't have.

The Usual Suspect, Ebola

Ebola was the original candidate for 'Disease X'. When epidemic Ebola actually broke out, it wasn't handled that way. It hadn't been formally transferred from a list of ultra-dangerous global security threats to those counting as African medical humanitarian emergencies, but informally that is what happened.[90] The 2014 outbreak of Ebola in west Africa didn't qualify as a pandemic in two respects. First – as correctly anticipated by the WHO and the CDC – it didn't spread across continents. Second, the virus wasn't new. It was already known to biomedicine, epidemiology, and anthropology. But the 2014 Ebola outbreak was more than just another epidemic. The story of Ebola in west Africa is a microcosm of the models and narratives of pandemic response and the hierarchy of knowledge. It was a new, disruptive, and frightening societal event. It showed how we need *both* emergency outbreak response *and* stronger health systems, and that they need to gel. The 'war on disease' script was invoked to reassure the people of the affected countries and the wider world – including the international media and political leaders in Europe and America, who were frightened it would travel to their countries. This script meant much of what was already known about how to contain Ebola's spread was ignored and had to be relearned.

The medical community knew more about Ebola than it realized. By the time he left Zaïre in December 1976, Peter Piot had not only shared in the virological triumph of isolating the pathogen, but he had done some anthropology too: working out the two main contexts in which the virus was transmitted. One was health care itself. The sisters of the mission in Yambuku bonded with the young Belgian doctor over their shared backgrounds in the villages around Antwerp and their commitment to saving the lives of the stricken people of the villages around Yambuku.

The nuns were totally committed women. They were brave. They faced an incredibly difficult environment and they dealt with it as best they could. They meant well. We had shared their table and their lives for what seemed like far longer than four days, and every evening, as they sipped their little tots of vermouth, they had told us about the villages of their childhoods. Every evening the discussion had ended up circling around and around the same subject – the epidemic. Who had fallen ill first, when it happened, and how. The dread of infection, the horrible deaths of their patients and colleagues. They had been trying to map out the frightening terrain until, I suppose, it would seem more manageable, less horrific. It was a narrative in which they had felt like heroes of a sort, and certainly martyrs.[91]

However, all those years earlier, Piot had discovered that their unsterilized needles had been an important element in the outbreak.

Now it appeared that they were in some sense villains as well. It was very hard to formulate the words that would inform the sisters that the virus had in all likelihood been amplified and spread by their own practices and lack of proper training. In the end I think we were far too polite about it: I'm not certain at all that it really sank in when we told them our preliminary conclusions.[92]

One of the hardest things for humanitarians to admit is that they are harming people. Time and again, visitors to relief programmes or health clinics in desperately poor parts of the world are shocked by what seems so obvious: that foreign aid workers are wilfully blind to the harms that they are doing. Aid workers' self-esteem is based on doing good, so that doing harm to harmless people simply doesn't fit. Psychologists call it cognitive dissonance. Individuals who are in this situation adopt psychological stratagems for protecting their image of themselves as good people. They may deny that they are acting voluntarily (the rules are set), or refuse to deal candidly with death (something commonplace in western societies), or attribute disagreeable traits to the victims (ranging from hostility to simple ignorance). Mary Douglas would have not been surprised: where matters of life and death are concerned, it's best to let the institution do the thinking.

The Yambuku sisters probably never fully accepted their culpability. Piot didn't need to draw attention to their lapses as the dangers of unsterilized needles were well known. Cases of infection through contaminated equipment do still occur occasionally and are probably more common than health workers like to admit. The bigger problem is that health professionals rarely look beyond the perimeter of their own compounds and appreciate how their simply being there can be a hazard.

Take the common situation of a small, under-equipped clinic in a poor rural district in west Africa. Its staff faithfully follow the basic procedures for sterilizing needles and have standard-issue gloves and face masks. Imagine that there's an outbreak of Ebola nearby. We know that a clinic can't do much for a patient who has Ebola beyond the most rudimentary treatment of keeping the individual hydrated. We know that the virus is extremely contagious, and that every step of the way from home to hospital bed presents a danger of infecting others. Travelling to a clinic in a taxi or bus, or being carried by bicycle or wheelbarrow; sitting or lying on the veranda of the health centre waiting to be seen by a nurse and a doctor, and then lying stricken in a ward with either a family member as a carer or an overworked assistant nurse cleaning up vomit, faeces and blood – these are ideal environments for contagion.

So why should a person sick with suspected Ebola actually go to a hospital? If she doesn't have Ebola, she has a high risk of contracting it from someone who does. If she does have it, she will probably die anyway. In a fairer world than ours in the early 21st century, African countries would have sanitized ambulances for safe transport of desperately sick patients and health centres would have the equipment and trained staff needed to treat them. But they don't. And patients still come, and nurses and doctors still treat them at terrifying risk to themselves, and to their families and co-workers. Why? Because that's just what they do. From a sense of expectation, of duty, of habit that somehow obscures risk, patients and health care workers carry out their everyday activities without apparent rational calculus of the danger. The institution carries on thinking for the individual.

If the patient dies in an Ebola treatment centre, she will die alone and be buried in a mass grave without being returned to her family for a respectful ceremony. This is a bad death, worse than death itself. For practitioners of western biomedicine, the relationship between doctor and patient ends when the patient dies. Despite the awareness of some physicians and psychologists about the importance of treating the end of life with sensitivity and respect, the routine way of treating a dead patient is as a problem to be disposed of. But relationships continue after death; there is unfinished business to be resolved. In many cultures, the afterlife is an unquestioned reality. In many African belief systems, the deceased person may be elevated to the standing of an ancestor spirit. When researchers noted that funerals were becoming *more* elaborate and expensive at the height of southern Africa's AIDS epidemic, despite the cost to the bereaved families, the answer emerged that because dying from AIDS was a bad death – premature, ugly, and from a stigmatized disease – the family needed to put extra effort into the transition to the next life.[93]

Understanding dying is important for containing Ebola. It's not something that people will talk about unless approached in a sympathetic way. Piot spent a lot of time listening and learning. He writes:

> I put together a picture of what happened during funerals. As in so many cultures, funerals were a major event for the Buja, stretching across several days and could easily cost a

full year's income. What made these funerals so lethal, apart
from the prolonged and intense contact, was the prepara-
tion of the cadaver. The body was thoroughly cleaned, and
the process often involved several family members, working bare-handed. Since the bodies were usually covered in
blood, feces and vomit, exposure to the Ebola virus was
enormous – particularly since the usual custom was to clean
all the orifices: mouth, eyes, nose, vagina, anus.[94]

A year after Piot published his memoir, Ebola fever broke
out in west Africa, initially in Guinea and spreading to the
neighbouring countries of Liberia and Sierra Leone. It killed
at least 12,000 people, probably more. Piot's virological
breakthrough back in 1976 was universally acknowledged
but his anthropological insights into transmission through
health care provision and during funerals were rediscovered
only when the epidemic was waning. Why? Because the
medical institutions did the thinking.

The patient zero was a young child in Guinea, probably
infected by playing under a tree where bats were roosting.
The initial outbreak appeared for a while to have been contained, but one infected person had crossed the border to
Sierra Leone. Cases exploded in that country's third largest town, Kenema. Public health experts feared that in the
overcrowded and unsanitary shanty towns of Sierra Leone
and Liberia, Ebola would spread unchecked. By August/
September 2014, the number of cases was doubling every
three weeks. Epidemiological models predicted uncontrolled
spread throughout west Africa causing more than a million
deaths, with the virus likely reaching Europe and America.[95]

Ebola was the number one disease on the list of the usual
suspects for a dangerous outbreak and therefore not a surprise. The WHO didn't respond – its leadership was busy
with its broader health agenda – but the system worked
insofar as others did, and the emergency reaction went
right to the very summit of global decision-making. On 18
September, the UN Security Council passed resolution 2177,

the first ever in response to a fast-breaking infectious disease emergency, declaring the epidemic a threat to international peace and security. China played its part. It sent aid for both emergency medicine and reconstruction, which it presented as south–south cooperation and a display of its growing influence in world politics.[96] China voted for resolution 2177, in what appears at first sight to be an uncharacteristic acceptance of health as an international security issue. Closer examination shows why the Chinese government was ready to go along with this. First, it was following the lead of African states which supported the resolution. Second, the text of the resolution emphasized that countries shouldn't close their borders or restrict travel unnecessarily. Most importantly, it framed the securitized response as an ad hoc decision by the UN Security Council – where China holds a veto – rather than making it the prerogative of the WHO. In summary, it kept the Ebola response safely insulated in its African humanitarian box.

The UN set up its Mission for Emergency Ebola Response (UNMEER), a specialized mission to support governments and international agencies. President Barack Obama dispatched the 101st Airborne to Liberia, the first ever deployment of a US army combat unit to 'fight' a disease – a war on 'warre' in what had been the epicentre of the feared 'coming anarchy'. This was part of the Pentagon's ever-expanding portfolio of responsibilities in post-9/11 America, where 'everything became war and the military became everything'.[97] The British government sent troops to Sierra Leone under a typically opaque acronym, the Joint Inter-Agency Task Force (JIATF).

Oliver Johnson, a physician at King's College London's Centre for Global Health, was working in Sierra Leone, where his clinic was turned over to the care of Ebola patients. The account that he co-wrote with Sinead Walsh (Ireland's ambassador to Sierra Leone) is a candid memoir of what was done right and what went wrong. Johnson was frustrated by just how slowly the international response was moving and was now disappointed that the military intervention wasn't the one that the doctors had been calling for. He had a vision of military doctors in hazmat suits running hospitals. But the British soldiers arrived under strict orders 'to ensure a "zero casualty rate" – among themselves – and their priority was "force protection". While they were often out and about during the day at various field sites, under no circumstances could the soldiers get too close to the Ebola frontline.'[98] They also brought military language. Sinead Walsh describes an encounter between Bintou Keita, a veteran of UNICEF who had a career's worth of experience in health care, who had been appointed to run UNMEER, and a British military officer, newly arrived, whom she tactfully doesn't name. The officer 'gave a presentation full of military language, like "attacking" the "enemy" of Ebola and maintaining a "battle rhythm" going after "escapees" from quarantine. Bintou sat quietly, writing down every military reference. She then took the official aside and showed him her notepad. She didn't have to say anything – he got the message and, after that, changed his tone.'[99]

Some people – myself included – mocked the military operations as an inordinately expensive public relations exercise that contributed little and distorted priorities.[100] From the accounts written by those in the field – such as those by Walsh and Johnson – this is unfair. Despite their high profile, the soldiers weren't actually running the show and were generally sensitive to the priorities of civilians, and their presence – especially their Medevac capacity – made it easier for international medical agencies to send staff to run programmes.[101]

The problem lies elsewhere, in the consensus that the biomedical response is what counts. Paul Farmer, one of the most politically progressive physician-advocates of our era, shows this in action. Over his career, in Haiti, in Boston, and around the world, Farmer has made a reputation as a critic of health care inequities and author of devastating exposés of the structural violence embedded in the world's capitalist system. A medical anthropologist, he has long insisted on culturally appropriate programmes.[102] Like most doctors, he hadn't prior experience with Ebola, but he knew enough. Farmer flew to Liberia in September 2014 just as the Ebola epidemic curve was bending upwards at its steepest. He wrote a passionate denunciation of the shocking under-investment in health care in west Africa, declaring: 'Ebola is more a symptom of a weak healthcare system than anything else.'[103] Returning to a long-standing theme in his writings, he added: '[T]he Ebola crisis should serve as an object lesson and rebuke to those who tolerate anaemic state funding of, or even cutbacks in, public health and healthcare delivery. Without staff, stuff, space and systems, nothing can be done.' He was specific:

> First, we need to stop transmission. ... [I]n the absence of an effective medical system, it occurs wherever care is given: in households, clinics and hospitals, and where the dead are tended. Infection control must be strengthened in all of these places, and during burials, which requires not only training and exhortations (which are already given in cities throughout West Africa, on billboards and radio, and in community meetings) but also uninterrupted supplies of personal protective equipment. Community health workers, too, need to be better equipped, trained and paid if they are to play a role in contact-tracing and early diagnosis, as well as trying to address the mounting number of deaths caused by other conditions.[104]

This is all correct, morally and empirically. It joins the health systems and the outbreak prevention agendas. But 'must' implies 'can'. Where 'staff, stuff, space and systems' couldn't reach, these calls to action weren't relevant, but things *could* still be done. Let's take one example from Walsh and Johnson's account. It should be obvious that it was safer to have patients cared for at home rather than bringing them to overcrowded hospitals. The best response to this would have been to provide personal protective equipment (PPE) and basic instructions for care to communities. But the officials responsible for the PPE supplies worried that they couldn't guarantee the proper use of PPE outside clinics, or ensure standards of care in places where they had no direct supervision, so this was never done.[105] The logic is to pretend not to see the problem over which we have no control.

The twin failing is playing down the risks of our own interventions. Many cases of Ebola were contracted at health facilities. Health workers died. Walsh spoke to a nurse in Kenema who said:

> I remember when the first patient came to Kenema. She was in the minor theatre. I was one of the first nurses, we were eight. We were told that it was very infectious, but I volunteered. Four of those nurses are dead and four are alive. Then in the second batch we were fifteen nurses, out of these seven are alive.[106]

In Kenema town alone, 80 health workers died. In the whole country, 221 health workers died, about 7 per cent of the entire health workforce.[107] They were heroes and martyrs. It is too painful to think that they might have been better advised to tell Ebola patients to stay at home. Beyond the perimeter of medical institutions' reach, some communities were improvising and learning and managing the epidemic just as well. To be exact, it was mostly women who were most vulnerable to the disease, and overwhelmingly women who led the response.[108] A team headed by Melissa Parker of the London School of Hygiene and Tropical Medicine investigated what happened in the remote village of Mathaineh, where there weren't Ebola clinics.[109] What they found was that communities were quick to learn the basics of the disease. People preferred to treat patients close to home and set up places in the nearby bush where they could be isolated from the rest of the community, with just one appointed carer. They were fed pepper soup and drank water with lime and honey. Local teams made home-made PPE. Although the statistics aren't conclusive because of the small numbers, the data show that this wasn't any worse than the formal response and probably was better. Out of 39 people cared for in this way, 27 survived.

The biggest problem that these Sierra Leonean communities faced was the coercive government response. People who failed to report Ebola cases were liable to be fined. The chief of a neighbouring village might report to the authorities that his counterpart wasn't cooperating with the official effort, to gain reward. The higher-up authorities might send in the troops to deal with a 'lawless' place 'unwilling to accept orders'.[110] This was a common problem. At an early stage of the epidemic, the government in next-door Liberia sent troops to isolate West Point, a large shanty town in the capital Monrovia. It was a fiasco: a violent confrontation between troops and residents followed. President Ellen Johnson-Sirleaf quickly reversed her decision and adopted a consensus-building approach. Back in Sierra Leone, the president declared a state of emergency and used soldiers and police officers to enforce (brutally) quarantine measures on a house-to-house basis. For residents, checkpoints and neighbourhood patrols reminded them of the war years.[111] It didn't work, partly because the soldiers were easy to bribe, partly because the lockdown imprisoned entire families and deprived them of food, water, and other basics. A later assessment estimated that Sierra Leone's lockdown probably prolonged the epidemic by as much as six months.[112]

Why did the authorities take this approach? Because that's what they do – perhaps it's the only thing they *can* do. To demonstrate its authority to its people and to its foreign aid donors, a weak government sends soldiers and police officers to do something visible and intrusive. Anthropologists call this the 'performative' state.

Farmer concluded his article with the words, 'Less palaver, more action.'[113] He meant fewer and shorter meetings among international aid donors. Most of the experts involved in the Ebola response would have agreed. But palaver with the local people, who are affected by the problem, is *never* a waste of time, even at the height of an emergency. It's a lesson that emergency aid givers learn in every disaster – and fail to apply in the next one. Walsh and Johnson conclude their book: 'The number one lesson we need to take from the Ebola crisis is the importance of good community engagement from the very beginning of a response.'[114]

The social anthropologist Paul Richards has spent 40 years in Sierra Leone, starting with studying what he calls the 'people's science' of agriculture. He was called upon to advise in the response to Ebola, initially because health policy experts wanted to know what harmful local traditions needed to be extirpated and how best to communicate expert knowledge.[115] Richards turned this task around, making the case that it was better to find out how communities and epidemiologists could learn from one another to develop a joint approach. Epidemiology, Richards says, is also a 'people's science'. He found that people well understood the dangers of getting infected at health centres and he emphasized the cultural importance of not dying alone and respecting funeral rites.[116]

Although, as noted above, in September 2014, when the epidemic was doubling every two to three weeks, the expectation was that it would kill over a million; in fact, it peaked and declined. There were 28,000 confirmed cases in the three adjoining countries (Guinea, Liberia, and Sierra Leone) plus isolated ones in Senegal and Nigeria. The official death toll was just under 12,000. The decline was more rapid and more widespread than expected and occurred before most of the international resources arrived. Most post-epidemic reviews focus on the international response, less so on what actually ended the epidemic.[117] Parker and her colleagues write:

> Many claims have been made about what was significant. These include effective partnerships between national/international armed forces and [international non-governmental organizations]; improvements in biomedical

therapy; increasingly effective political leadership; rolling out community care centres; contributions from paramount chiefs; and local learning. All these factors may have been important at different times, and in different places, but there is a paucity of evidence.[118]

The evidence is poor because the researchers didn't look for it. Following Richards, it appears that the medical establishment rediscovered Piot's lessons about Ebola after having tried everything else first. The response was important, but more important was what communities did, either on their own or in discussions with health experts. Post hoc modelling of the epidemic trajectory shows that the best simulation of the decline in transmission is based on the widespread adoption of a community-based strategy for screening and restricting movement. The author of this assessment concludes, 'We know of no other similarly validated explanation for the end of the outbreak.'[119] This is also recognized in the declassified US National Security Council report on the epidemic: 'Transmission rates in Liberia fell far faster than predicted, with community behavior and social mobilization emerging as more potent factors in stopping Ebola than the build out of isolation and treatment facilities at the core of the initial strategy.'[120] That's a lesson worth dwelling on: security advisers in the White House acknowledged that the need for community involvement in regular health care also applied to emergency epidemic response. It confirms Richards' wider conclusion, noted in the opening chapter, that people change their practices if approached in the right spirit: 'It is striking how rapidly communities learnt to think like epidemiologists, and epidemiologists to think like communities.'[121]

6

Emancipatory Catastrophe? Covid-19

We were warned. Repeatedly and in detail. 'There is a very real threat of a rapidly moving highly lethal pandemic of a respiratory pathogen killing 50 to 80 million people and wiping out nearly 5% of the world's economy. . . . The world is not prepared.'[1] Those words were written in September 2019 by Gro Harlem Brundtland and Elhadj As Sy,[2] who jointly chaired the WHO's Global Preparedness Monitoring Board (GPMB). Indeed, anyone tasked with writing a post mortem on the Covid-19 pandemic could save a lot of time and effort by simply reprinting any one of several reports on pandemic preparedness published before it happened, and checking off each warning and each recommendation. The summary would be a column of checks each reading 'ignored' or 'told you so'. In their September 2020 report, Brundtland and Sy wrote, 'Never before has the world been so clearly forewarned of the dangers of a devastating pandemic, nor previously had the knowledge, resources and technologies to deal with such a threat.'[3]

United Nations organizations employ ghost writers with the special skill of watering down phrases, using the passive voice, choosing don't-offend-anyone turns of phrase, and using simple easy-to-translate sentences. The pre-Covid-19 GPMB report is a compelling read all the same. Even more precisely prescient is a background paper from Johns Hopkins that focuses on respiratory pathogens other than influenza – a category that includes Covid-19.[4] Every challenge was known in advance. Many countries had developed the infrastructure for rapid testing and diagnosis and played out scenarios to respond, often with technical assistance from the CDC in Atlanta. In Washington, DC, itself, the bipartisan Commission on Strengthening America's Health Security formulated a package of recommendations in November 2019.[5] One thing that they all stressed was that preparedness was a good investment. For less than $40 billion ($5 per person per year), the world could have been spared an estimated $21 trillion in the costs and losses of Covid-19.[6]

One of the themes of this book is that pandemic pathogens are surprises to science and society. This wasn't the case for the virus SARS-CoV-2. Important details weren't known, but these all fell within the ambit of what we could call the *normal uncertainties*. Virologists sequenced the genome of SARS-CoV-2 within weeks, publicizing their findings and exploring familiar and novel vaccine technologies. Physicians made rapid progress in learning the spectrum of symptoms and what and what not to do to treat it. Epidemiologists began with fewer datapoints to project its spread and their models (drawn from influenza) needed major adjustments as the pandemic unfolded. This was all as expected. Public health experts had prepared a playbook for responses, which included how best to communicate with the public, ensure that poor countries and poor communities had adequate resources to respond, and that 'whole of government' and 'whole of society' strategies were followed, an approach that (in the words of the GPMB) included 'community engagement': 'It is essential to understand community needs and ensure their systematic incorporation into planning and accountability mechanisms.'[7] The GPMB doesn't go deep into what 'accountability' means beyond reporting back to WHO committees and participating in post-pandemic evaluations. But there's a sting in the word: we must blame political leaders as well as pathogens.

Experts in infectious diseases had been worried about the radical uncertainties of a new pathogen. It turned out that the science had so improved in the years since SARS that the uncertainties were well within the scope of the anticipated. The radical uncertainty was in the politics – something that none of the experts had thought to anticipate. SARS-CoV-2 is a politically sophisticated pathogen, whose impact lies more in what it does to the body politic than what it does to the human body. The politics of response to Covid-19 was a disorienting combination. The political right invited popular debate on public health expertise, in pursuit of its new-found agenda of disrupting institutions. In the name of free-thinking, agitators veered into pseudo-science and conspiracy theories. Liberals and the left valorized scientists and rushed to embrace a standardized set of suppression measures. Lockdowns were over-engineered and had momentous social and economic consequences; some critics detected authoritarian longings.[8]

Covid-19 is more deadly than seasonal flu, but much less so than SARS or 1918 influenza, let alone the fearsome maximally malignant (monster) virus. Its speciality is a feature that the virologist-designed MMMV lacked, namely parasitizing on our most essential social and economic activities, so that we can't suppress it without making our societies seize up too. The Covid-19 *crisis* is at least as big as the pandemic – we need that old word 'pandemy' back.

As I write this in December 2020, it's far too early in the Covid-19 pandemic to tell its story. No judgements can be made about which policies worked and which didn't until it is over. In this final chapter, I will instead provide a brief tour of the disordered world under the coronavirus and then turn to three questions. The first of these begins with the biggest loser – the United States – to ask: who gained from the disruption? The second question reprises the recurrent theme of the scientific paradigm shift that follows pandemics: where will we find ourselves if we follow the science? The last is: what kind of politics are needed?

De-Prepared

The world wasn't unprepared. A handful of world leaders had *de*-prepared. China and America had each weakened the pandemic response system, in different ways and for their different reasons.

The outbreak began in China in November 2019 and, as forewarned, China did as it had done before: a brief confusion followed by a relentless imposition of order. Here it is clear that the institutions did the thinking. President Xi Jinping wasn't going to repeat the political errors of SARS-CoV-1 in 2003 when China had lost control of the science, the politics, and the narrative. All the necessary levers of policy were now in his hands and he acted accordingly. His government strictly controlled information, suppressed independent reports, and covered up the fact that local authorities were incentivized to suppress bad news such as anomalous new diseases. China also had a containment plan which it acted upon. The government instructed scientists to accelerate their virological research. It shut down the city of Wuhan in January 2020 with the aim of eliminating person-to-person transmission of the virus. It consisted of low-tech isolation measures enforced by a pyramid of people's committees with disciplinary powers, combined with some high-technology electronic surveillance. Neighbourhood 'grids', organized to control migrants, meant that large numbers of local people could be switched to contact tracing and curfew enforcement. Locking down a city and surrounding area, with 56 million people, was a response without precedent and went far beyond the WHO recommendations. It was the kind of over-engineered response possible only in a ruthless authoritarian state, and it worked. Outside Wuhan, there were targeted measures such as closing schools and testing and contact tracing.

President Xi launched what he called a 'people's war' against Covid-19 and promised to lead the country to victory. Amid martial images, the state news agency Xinhua posted a video of him visiting Wuhan, entitled 'The People's Leader Commanding the Decisive Battle'.[9] The government's war, or, more correctly, its policing, was also directed to suppress an epidemic of derogatory and satirical commentary on social media.

China extended cooperation to the WHO, but only on its own terms. The Director General of the WHO was an Ethiopian, Dr Tedros Adhanom Ghebreyesus, who had been elected on his reputation as a highly capable health minister and an agreeable foreign minister. He found himself with vast responsibility and little power – precisely the position for which the previous 15 years' global health diplomacy had set him up. Tedros needed America or China to empower him. Neither did so. Instead, they bullied him. Tedros followed the book and followed China. He procrastinated a week before declaring a public health emergency of international concern – a long time in the epidemic's exponential growth phase. The WHO was trapped in the paradox of rule-bound emergency response: no formal procedure can dictate the rapid and creative action that is needed to snatch solutions in the moment. The US government, tracking the new disease using its own monitoring capacity, could have energized the WHO. In fact, the new dispensation relied on America doing so. President Trump had no regard for conventional protocols and a single phone call to Tedros would have sufficed – or a tweet such as: COVID THE WORST PANDEMIC IN A HUNDRED YEARS; ACT NOW!! But the Trump administration saw the WHO as an alien entity rather than an instrument for the mutual needs of America and the rest of the world. The United Nations Secretary General was forced to be spectator rather than statesman, his microphone muted while China and America bickered. In March, many countries demanded that the UN Security Council take the minimum step of making a statement. China insisted that the disease fell outside the Council's geo-political ambit (unlike its position on Ebola). The United States insisted that any Security Council statement mention that the virus originated in China. There was no statement.

The first case outside China was diagnosed in Thailand in January, by scientists who had been trained as part of the global preparedness efforts. Thailand dutifully followed the WHO–CDC playbook. So too did other countries in East and South-east Asia. Their responses and patterns of infection varied: each had its own tradition of public health and policing, its own infrastructure for housing, public transport, markets, factories, and offices, and its own intimate social behaviours. People usually greet one another through bowing, rather than embracing and kissing on the cheek, and readily wear face masks. Most countries had also been studious partners in American-led preparedness planning. South Korea's President Moon Jae-in declared 'war' on the coronavirus and his government followed a strategy based on a centrally directed test–trace–isolate plan, enforced with harsh penalties. Taiwan, which had revised its preparedness after SARS, implemented a model response based on rigorous screening of arrivals, quarantining, and contact tracing, and avoided a shutdown. Central to its 'all of society' approach was transparent daily communication with the public.[10] In its earlier attempts to join the World Health Assembly, Taiwan had declared itself an indispensable front in the 'war on disease',[11] but martial metaphor was notably absent from its response to Covid-19. Singapore enforced a near-lockdown: it efficiently policed the virus, confining the major outbreaks to the dormitories where foreign workers lived.

Japan followed a haphazard approach, relying on good science and social conformity to keep transmission down in the 'three Cs' of confined indoor spaces, crowds, and close-contact settings. On the anniversary of Japan's defeat in

World War II, Emperor Naruhito used understated language: 'While we are currently confronted with the unprecedented difficulties caused by the spread of the coronavirus disease 2019, I sincerely hope that we all work together hand in hand to overcome this difficult situation and continue to seek happiness of the people and world peace.'[12]

Australia and New Zealand hoped geography would protect them, as with influenza a century earlier. They attempted protective sequestration for their whole countries, which kept the coronavirus out at first.

The virus reached Europe. The first cases were in northern Italy in January, in the cities of Lombardy, where the practice of policing epidemics was first formalized 600 years ago. The Italian government scaled the Wuhan experiment up to the first ever nationwide shutdown. The world had never seen anything like it. A comprehensive ban on movement and socialization will shut down transmission of any airborne infection, and so it did, for a while. Why Italy went to this extreme so fast isn't clear. Taiwan, South Korea, and everywhere in China outside Wuhan had used targeted 'find–test–trace–isolate' approaches, which were indeed the WHO's recommendations. The idea of a total shutdown could be found in influenza control models, but only as a theoretical point of reference – few experts on NPIs thought it would ever be workable in practice, and certainly not for longer than a month or so.[13] Still more unexpected was that the Italian experiment became the model for much of the world. In China, the rationale had been to eradicate transmission. In Europe, the aim was to 'flatten the curve': to reduce the number of people falling critically ill in the short term so that hospitals could cope. Buying time was also a chance to build the apparatus needed for WHO/Asian-style 'find–test–trace–isolate' containment. Most European governments, however, used the painfully secured delay to micro-engineer the lockdown measures themselves instead of constructing the containment system that would be needed when the lockdowns were lifted. Spain followed the

Italian model. So did France. For good measure, President Emmanuel Macron declared war on Covid-19, but not very convincingly. Germany had a different emphasis, on mass testing and contact tracing, confident that its hospitals could cope, and German Chancellor Angela Merkel avoided military language. Sweden relied on social conformism rather than administrative diktat. Commentators have been quick to judge these strategies as successes or failures based on the first few months – far too quickly.

Hungary's Viktor Orbán snapped up emergency powers, using the pandemic as a pretext to implement his authoritarian and xenophobic agenda. In Tsarist tradition, Russia's Vladimir Putin was more worried by political unrest than by the disease and put security officers in charge. Reviving the Soviet practice of treating technological progress as geostrategic rivalry, he christened Russia's experimental vaccine Sputnik V and declared it safe and available before it had been properly tested.

Britain had previously been a world leader in pandemic preparedness. Those who drew up the plans were worried that they had been neglected for some years. The plans also had a systemic defect: they had no contingencies for disruptive leadership. Prime Minister Boris Johnson briefly took the political stage as if he were a ghost from the 1830s, breezily dismissing containment measures as humbug before he reversed course in March and ordered a nationwide shutdown. Johnson's attempts to invoke the spirit of the Battle of Britain and declare himself head of a wartime government sounded hollow as he had used up that metaphorical stock over Brexit. There was a fierce debate in Britain over whether to follow the continental model or to aim for herd immunity – achieved when enough people have acquired immunity through infection or vaccination to stop general transmission of the virus. The herd immunity approach was drawn from models for influenza, which assumed a seasonal pattern with brief (two- to three-month) waves and a vaccine within a year. But no one knew whether Covid-19 would follow this script (it didn't), and because testing was haphazard and limited, no one had the slightest idea how many people had been infected so the case-fatality rate was no more than guesswork.[14] Into this blizzard of uncertainties stepped a team of epidemiological modellers at Imperial College London, led by Neil Ferguson. Given that their model was influential in government decision-making, it is worth quoting the short passage in which they candidly admit its limitations:

> It is important to note at the outset that given SARS-CoV-2 is a newly emergent virus, much remains to be understood about its transmission. In addition, the impact of many of the NPIs detailed here depends critically on how people respond to their introduction, which is highly likely to vary between countries and even communities. Last, it is highly likely that there would be significant spontaneous changes in population behaviour even in the absence of government-mandated interventions.[15]

Note that there are three different uncertainties contained in this single paragraph. One, 'much remains to be understood': the basic datapoints for sound epidemiology are not yet known. In short, it's *only* a model. Two, impact depends upon how people respond to the measures, which will vary. Three, there will be 'significant spontaneous changes in population behaviour' regardless of policy. In the debate that followed, points two and three were ignored entirely: the policy question was framed exclusively as herd immunity versus lockdown. In turn, lockdown was presented as 'flattening the curve' to 'defend the National Health Service'. There were alternatives. Britain could have learned from Taiwan that transparency works, from Japan, South Korea, and Germany that targeted interventions work as well as blanket ones, and from Sierra Leone that community mobilization is the best way of designing and implementing NPIs.

In the global south, the Covid-19 crisis arrived before the virus. African governments rushed to shut down their countries before they had outbreaks, because it appeared to be the international 'best practice'. They didn't ask what the shutdowns were supposed to achieve. It wasn't feasible to sequestrate countries entirely or to eliminate transmission, and the consequences for other health conditions, hunger, and livelihoods were catastrophic. No African health ministry could build up hospital capacity to cope with an expected surge of cases. No centralized all-of-government 'find–test–trace–isolate' mechanisms were feasible. It would have been possible to consult communities and find locally designed and locally monitored ways to re-plan markets, reconfigure public transport and schools to reduce transmission risks, and shield the most vulnerable (such as the elderly) from exposure. Forgetful of the hard-won lessons of recent epidemics, governments reverted to assuming that leaders knew best, even when it was self-evident that they were groping in the dark. South Africa adopted comprehensive restrictions and rolled out welfare payments to mitigate the hardship. It was an elaborate central plan drawn up for an imaginary country, without participation from communities and no insights from history or anthropology.[16] Notably, police and soldiers enforced bans on alcohol and bereaved families were forbidden from burying their dead according to custom. In the first weeks, this shut down the virus; by the end of the year, South Africa had the worst epidemic on the continent. The Kenyan authorities took the opportunity to accelerate slum clearances, making a mockery of the stay-at-home order by demolishing people's homes. There were two African outliers, Tanzania and Burundi, whose presidents insisted that faith in God would be sufficient to stop the virus. Burundi's President Pierre Nkurunziza died in June. In line with his Covid denialism in life, his death was officially attributed to a heart attack.

Latin American official responses spanned the spectrum from leftist populist denialism (Mexico) to far-right populist denialism (Brazil), with versions of Italian-style lockdowns (Argentina, Chile, and Peru) in-between. Jair Bolsonaro of Brazil portrayed the virus as a foreign threat demanding a military response, but did not turn that into a wider government mobilization against it. Others evoked the war metaphor in a half-hearted way. Everywhere the contours of sickness and deprivation followed racial and class divides, with indigenous and African-origin populations the worst hit. Ecuador suffered one of the world's worst epidemics early on, for reasons that have defied easy explanation, its toll surpassing the capacity of the state to count the dead.

India under Narendra Modi implemented a spectacular and misconceived performance of central state power in the form of a comprehensive shutdown on 24 March without a single day's prior warning. Tens of millions of workers in cities crammed onto buses and trains to return to their villages. This unleashed enormous economic hardship and signally and predictably failed to contain the virus. The state of Kerala stood out as an exception, drawing on its long-established model of social medicine, but as with too many other success stories, it relapsed later. Iran, which was hit hard early because it didn't pause its flights to China, admitted to a crisis and concealed a larger one. Syria, still in a long and ravaging civil war, gave up on any systematic response.

We heard a lot of martial language and grew used to military involvement in domestic public health. Many countries deployed soldiers to provide emergency hospital care and to enforce lockdowns. In some places, the army took control of health policy or used public health emergency powers for overtly repressive ends. Surveillance became normalized. For liberals, it is a disagreeable rediscovery that restrictive measures that limit migration, travel, and meeting in public, and intrusive monitoring of personal behaviour, are part of the campaign plan because they actually do restrict disease transmission. The conservative reactions were more unexpected.

Disruptive Capitalism and the Coronavirus

The novel coronavirus reached America from Europe. The country that had led the world in pandemic preparedness for 20 years was the most de-prepared of all. The United States followed a path all of its own. In the week of the election (3 November), the daily count of Covid-19 cases passed 100,000 and the country had suffered 231,000 deaths and the ignominy of surrendering its world leadership. The obvious culprit was Donald J. Trump himself, a germophobe who had dictated his personal health reports, but the deeper problem lay in the radical de-institutionalization of governance.

During 2020, Trump zigzagged. He started off by dismissing Covid-19 as a hoax and nothing worse than seasonal flu; advertised random treatments; flirted with the 'war leader' script; blamed China and the 'deep state'; made public health guidance a dividing line in the political culture wars and signalled to far-right vigilantes that they should 'liberate' Democrat-run states under quasi-lockdown; denounced leading scientists; adopted a macho defiance when he himself contracted the virus in October; before shifting back into fatalism about the uncontrolled spread of the virus in the final weeks before the election. Without leadership from Washington, DC, individual states and cities designed their own package measures. Most called it 'lockdown', but it was in fact a menu of travel restrictions, social distancing (more properly, physical distancing), closures of schools, restaurants, and workplaces, quarantine and contact tracing, and stay-at-home orders, unevenly decreed and inconsistently followed. Testing was chaotic, which meant that crucial data weren't available.

The president and his disciples made science partisan. Democrats lauded scientists while Republicans distrusted them. The head of the National Institute of Allergy and Infectious Diseases, Dr Anthony Fauci, became the lightning rod for whether politics should follow science, or science should bend to politics. Every uncertainty in the data, every vagary in the recommendations, became a crack levered open to cast aspersions on scientists' authority and even honesty. The White House Coronavirus Task Force consulted epidemiological modellers such as Chris Murray of the Institute for Health Metrics and Evaluation at the University of Washington but didn't follow his advice when it didn't suit them. For example, the White House urged that states should reopen in April when Murray's model said it was still unsafe to do so. The Federal Government became unwilling to release essential epidemiological data, perhaps because the science contradicted the president's optimistic prognoses. Liberal critics attacked Trump for his scientific illiteracy, indifference to other people's lives, and chaos. There was, however, method in his mayhem. Part of it was a well-tuned practice of trying out different improvised messages to see which ones got the right echo among his followers, and setting the headlines every week. The constant subtexts were celebrating the virtues of personal freedom in a capitalist nation (and protecting the stock market) along with a simple sincere faith that science would deliver a magic bullet (so that everything would be alright in the end).

We can trace this political doctrine back to Ayn Rand (1905–82), prophet of radical capitalism. According to Rand, the individual is entitled to live the life of his or her choice with limitless freedom heedless of others. The previous generation of neo-liberals had seen their task as holding back the tide of communism; Rand and her devotees took this a stage further and condemned as evil *any* restraints on freedom of capital. This is a charter for disruption, one anticipated by James Dale Davidson and William Rees-Mogg, who opened their disturbing and prescient book *The Sovereign Individual* at the turn of the millennium by quoting Tom Stoppard: 'The future is disorder. A door like this has cracked open five or six times since we got on our hind legs. It is the best possible time to be alive, when almost everything you thought you knew is wrong.'[17] Davidson and Rees-Mogg foresaw the combination of the information revolution and the freeing of financial capital from state regulation bringing a huge wave of creative destruction. They didn't just describe the coming turmoil, they *relished* it.

Disruption wrecks institutions, of both the legal-rational and the informal-societal kinds, and so is a chance for the talented, wealthy, and bold to rise further. An ungoverned society is, for them, a virtuous one. Davidson and Reed-Mogg depict persons of wealth metamorphosing into 'sovereign individuals' who 'achieve financial escape velocity' from the gravitational pull of deadweight social contracts in failing nation-states.[18] They don't concern themselves with public health; indeed radical capitalists see it as an oxymoron. Rand didn't seem to make any effort to understand public health, as shown by her throwaway line praising the industrial revolution for increasing life expectancy beyond 30 years: 'Anyone over 30 years of age today, give a silent "Thank you" to the nearest, grimiest, sootiest smokestacks you can find.'[19] Such a vision needs a sunny world compatible with the unlimited pursuit of happiness. Rand herself calls it the 'benevolent universe' premise.[20]

The Trump administration set out to dismantle or weaken every regulatory or scientific institution that it could, and that included the pandemic preparedness apparatus built by his predecessors, both Republican and Democrat. This included the CDC, USAID's Emerging Pandemic Threats Program, and institutions for gathering key population data from the Census Bureau downwards. National Security Advisor John Bolton disbanded the directorate for Global Health Security and Biodefense at the National Security Council in 2018, on the grounds of efficiency and to better focus on traditional military threats. At the time, the Washington, DC, online journal *Outside the Beltway* commented: 'This is monumentally stupid.'[21] But Bolton was not a stupid man, just a dogmatic one. His doctrine was that power needs no justification and should respect no constraint.

For today's disruptive radical capitalists, the turmoil of a pandemic should be turned to political, commercial, and ideological advantage. In this regard, there's a notable economic difference between historic pandemics and Covid-19. The plague, smallpox, and influenza killed in sufficient numbers to make labour scarce and therefore increase wages and workers' political bargaining power. It doesn't look likely that Covid-19 will do that. To the contrary, it is making unskilled labour redundant and intensifying the problem of people surplus to the demands of the market. Insofar as the market decides who gets vaccinated first, it will sharpen these inequalities. There are commercial winners too. Corporations with deep pockets, good credit ratings, and the ear of politicians who deliver financial aid packages are doing better than small family businesses that don't have any of these things. This helps explain the otherwise puzzling performance of the stock market: the winners are listed on the Dow Jones, not the losers. The big exception to this is fossil fuels, as the recession accelerates decarbonization. In electoral contests, politicians who disregard social distancing rules can energize their campaigns with rallies, while those who stick to those rules handicap themselves.

On the fringes of the alt-right, some see Covid-19 as a plot by deep state entities to serve some devilish agenda, and on the fringes of those fringes there are probably some who follow the thinking of Adolf Hitler, who in *Mein Kampf* wrote approvingly of plague as a force for cleansing population and society.[22] Tolerating the conspiracist fringe is the cost of libertarian dogma and has also had tactical advantages in disrupting the establishment consensus in the public sphere.

Trump used military language only briefly. This is a puzzle easily solved. It would have entrapped him. Trump was a specialist in political theatre who honed the art of inciting and licensing factional violence but shied away from any real wars. War leaders use unifying scripts to rally their nations. They submit their decision-making to the institutionalized rigours of command and control, in which authority is matched with accountability. These were anathema to Trump. He shifted the fight to a territory and style more favourable to him: inflaming America's culture war over face masks and lockdowns and continuing his combative political business as usual.

Radical capitalists make *everything* a commodity that can be bought and sold in a market. The natural wilderness, the deep sea, the surface of the moon, the building blocks of life, endangered species, our human attention and everyday social interactions, public information – everything is tradable. The reason for making something into a commodity is that it can be owned by a person or a corporation and transacted for profit. Political power becomes commodified too. I call this the 'political market', in which power is broken down into its quanta – personal allegiances, laws, public media, security services, sovereign powers – which are bought and sold on a competitive basis according to the laws of supply and demand.[23] The beauty of this doctrine is that its practitioners don't need to understand it in order to master it. It follows a simple logic whereby transactional deal-making – political business as usual – trumps laws and institutions. This produces results in everyday politics and – to the frustration of politicians who invest in science, public goods, and a sustainable future – it also thrives in times of disorder. Transactional-charismatic leaders like Trump have learned their craft through practice, not study or strategic calculation, but it works. The media owned by Rupert Murdoch and other Randians treat news and opinion as commodities and audiences as markets. They have refined the practice of commodifying and marketing the public realm. Their content promotes these doctrines too, but plutocratic populists today are less interested in what the masses think and say, provided that the political market decides the political winner.

Radical capitalists have a naïve faith in a forgiving natural world. In one of those accidents of evolution that mimic intelligent design, SARS-CoV-2 hit on a sociology of transmission that exploited the circuits of the globalized economy and the faultlines of the transactional political marketplace. The novel coronavirus isn't the nemesis of radical capitalism – the two parasitize on one another's disruptive politics.

What Is It Like to Be a Bat (Virus)?

In previous chapters, I have anthropomorphized the microbial protagonists; not so the novel coronavirus SARS-CoV-2. Others will certainly portray it as a character – more surreptitious and cunning than its older cousin SARS-CoV-1. More has been discovered about this virus in the short period after the first cases of atypical pneumonia were diagnosed in Wuhan than for any other pathogen in history, with commensurate advances in diagnostics, treatments, and the development of vaccines. My question here is: what are the deeper paradigm shifts underway in scientific thinking?

The philosopher Thomas Nagel wrote a well-known essay entitled 'What Is It Like to Be a Bat?'[24] It was a thought experiment that questioned the coherence of materialist reductionist theories of consciousness and our intuitions about the workings of the world. Nagel chose bats because we accept that they have experiences but their sensory perception is sufficiently different to ours – they use echolocation to navigate – that we find it hard but not impossible to try to think like them. As we try to switch from our species-specific viewpoint, we can just about imagine what it would be like to have a mental map of space generated by echolocation. A few blind children have actually acquired that skill.

Nagel's argument is more relevant than the happenstance of his choice of subject. It's about how scientists' intuition is refined as scientific paradigms develop, and the gap that opens up between the scientists' understanding of the world and our everyday appreciation of it. Research virologists develop not only scientific insight but also intuition:

they learn to think like the pathogens – to be more exact, to have a mental model of how microbes function that goes beyond the formulae specified in their academic papers. It's an imaginary that allows scientists to make sense of statements that describe aspects of the world far outside our immediate experience. This isn't some post-modernist relativism, it is *real* discovery, just as the planets found by astronomers are real things. The point is that as scientific frameworks develop, so too scientists refine their intuitions. Nagel gives an example from Einstein's physics, the statement that 'matter is energy'. This is something we are taught at school that doesn't conform with our lived experience. (Newtonian physics is closer.) But physicists have integrated Einstein's general relativity into their cognitive processes, which is why they can use those theories to discover real planets. Laypeople who haven't developed this specialist literacy must take their statements on trust, in much the same way as they would a 'truth' revealed by a religious authority. Nagel writes, 'This explains the magical flavor of popular presentations of fundamental scientific discoveries, given out as propositions to which one must subscribe without really understanding them.'[25] Note, however, that the meaning of 'truth' is slippery here: for the theoretical physicist, 'truth' is the best hypothesis and is always open to refinement or falsification – the comfort of 'truthiness' lies in the credibility of scientific method, not in the findings as they exist today. It's different to the everyday 'truth' in which grass is green. Truth really does depend on what the meaning of 'is' is.[26]

Charlatans and denialists make the elementary category mistake (some deliberately so) of assuming that doubt or indeterminacy at one level of scientific explanation casts doubt on all scientific discoveries. Some are flat earthers; all have a flat epistemology of science.

The word 'virus' itself has evolved as biomedical science has deepened its understanding: from an inanimate poison; to an inferred microbial agent too small to be seen through an optical microscope; to an infective agent that requires a host cell to be able to multiply; to 'a statistical consensus of a genetically heterogenous population in a state of constant flux'.[27] Viruses don't readily submit to our taxonomies. As methods for identifying them have become more exact, the indeterminacies have become both more precise and more fundamental.

Can we imagine what it means to be a virus? It's only meaningful to think of what it is 'like' to be a virus insofar as it's possible to think of what it is 'like' to be a process of the survival of the fittest in a changing ecology. To adapt Louis Pasteur, microbial evolution will have the last word.[28] This means seeing diseases as the intersection of host, agent, and environment.

Let's start with the original host. There are more than 1,200 bat species in the world, adding up to almost a fifth of all mammal species. One reason for this profusion is that they diverged early from the rest of the mammalian family tree. Another is that they fly, which allows them to find diverse ecologies with different food sources and adapt accordingly. Bats host many different kinds of viruses which have only recently been researched.[29] It's possible that flying puts such demands on mammalian physiology that their immune systems are accommodating to viruses. Because bats roost in densely packed colonies and then disperse widely, intermingling with bats from other colonies, they sustain intersecting webs of viral transmission. Today, bat numbers are dwindling as forests are cut down. Species that thrive are those that can adapt to living on farms, on plantations, and in urban areas. In turn, they change how they roost and where they fly, leading to new patterns of viral transmission among bats and more chances for spillover to other animals.[30]

Humans and domesticated livestock constitute 96 per cent of the terrestrial mammalian biomass today.[31] Never in evolutionary history has a tiny range of large animal species at the top of the food chain been so dominant. Our factory-farmed pigs, cattle, and poultry are huge in number but extremely narrow in genetic diversity. Viruses have adapted to epochal transformations since the beginnings of multi-cellular life. With an evolutionary speed a million times faster than mammals, any microbe that can insert itself into mammalian cells has stumbled into a new world of an immense susceptible population – naïve hosts, in the revealing specialist term.

A generation of microbiologists have been warning us that if we want to keep our current way of life, we must constantly stay ahead of pathogens' evolution. Evolutionary biologists call this the 'Red Queen' dynamic, after the character in *Alice through the Looking Glass* who tells Alice she must run as fast as she can to stay in the same place. The microbiology of the Anthropocene suggests this metaphor is under-powered: we must *accelerate* as fast as we can to keep up with the quickening pace of microbial mutation and zoonotic spillover. Sustaining our hyperdominance requires an ever more elaborate engineering of the planetary environment, from climate to viruses. If we see our other lifeforms as either our possessions or our enemies, we have set ourselves on waging a war, which evolutionary logic tells us we cannot win. Such a historical ecological paradigm was once a minority view among infectious disease specialists. No longer. The concept of 'One Health' is gaining acceptance. This is the notion that the health of the planet, animal life, and human beings are interlinked. We need to understand the intersecting dynamics of pathogens, the environment, veterinary health, public health, and human livelihoods, and act in a joined-up way, fast.

This is the refined intuition of research scientists today. Reflecting on 'how we got to Covid-19', two of the world's most respected virologists, David Morens and Anthony Fauci, wrote:

> Science will surely bring us many life-saving drugs, vaccines, and diagnostics; however, there is no reason to think that these alone can overcome the threat of ever more frequent and deadly emergences of infectious diseases. . . . The COVID-19 pandemic is yet another reminder, added to

the rapidly growing archive of historical reminders, that in a human-dominated world, in which our human activities represent aggressive, damaging, and unbalanced interactions with nature, we will increasingly provoke new disease emergences. We remain at risk for the foreseeable future. COVID-19 is among the most vivid wake-up calls in over a century. It should force us to begin to think in earnest and collectively about living in more thoughtful and creative harmony with nature, even as we plan for nature's inevitable, and always unexpected, surprises.[32]

To think like a bat virus is to think like an evolutionary algorithm in a disrupted environment populated by a host of naïve hosts. If we think of microbiologists as explorers, what they are reporting is not that the novel coronavirus should be a new island to add to the map, but that we need an entirely new atlas. Covid-19 is the first malignant monster of our Anthropocene.

Alternatives to the 'War on Disease'

The time for the war on infectious disease has passed. It is a set of old metaphors that have rotted away and become layers of sediment on the bed of the river. When we kick them up, we just muddy the water; we stop thinking critically at the critical moment.

The idea of a war on disease served as a way of organizing thinking and action that allowed public leaders to act in the middle of intersecting uncertainties. It was a consensus across the political range that provided a comforting narrative at a time of fear. Its particular value was that it allowed us to anticipate a victorious homecoming. In the time of Covid-19, the striking thing about political narratives is how little the 'war' story has done for anyone. Xi Jinping has been most consistent and conventional in trying to instrumentalize the martial script. A number of aspiring authoritarians tried to follow the Hungarian path of taking emergency powers, but citizens have been vigilant about this ploy. Many countries rescheduled elections, but only Abiy Ahmed in Ethiopia postponed national elections without setting a new date. Intriguingly, right-wing authoritarians such as Bolsanaro, Modi, and Trump avoided picking a fight with the virus and used fighting language only to appear macho and to vilify groups or countries they didn't like. The WHO's GPMB hasn't mentioned 'war', 'fighting', or 'victory' over disease at all.

What will happen when governments around the world reconstruct pandemic preparedness and prevention? The first post-Covid-19 reviews have begun by lamenting the missed opportunities.[33] That's justifiable, but global health experts are also well aware of the limitations of their proposed mechanisms. The response to today's pandemic merges with vigilance against the next one, anticipated to be worse.[34] While we build new global public health institutions, we must be mindful that there's no global health solution to global health crises. As Morens and Fauci observed, vaccines don't address the underlying drivers of the risks. To the contrary, engineering our species' immunity to new pathogens as they arise, at warp speed, may be a dangerous triumph that indulges a misplaced faith in a safe homecoming return to 'normality'. There is no comfort in the status quo ante. Scientists and literate citizens know that we need urgent, far-reaching, and informed change. Could it be that, as we stare into the abyss, we decide to let go of the mental handrail that has guided us to the precipice, with an illusion of safety at every step?

Could Covid-19 become what Ulrich Beck called an 'emancipatory catastrophe'?[35] If so, what would be a new, emancipatory narrative for what we do about pandemic diseases, actual and threatened? I suggest that we begin with a return to a word introduced in chapter 1, and left waiting in the wings: 'pandemy'. As our leading scientists insist, pandemic disease is too important to be left to the biomedical establishment. It's a crisis in our way of life. In using the word 'pandemy', we can reclaim the concept of a holistic disruption, reaching backwards into the ecological, social, and health pathologies that have created virulent pathogens with pandemic potential, broadening to include other illnesses prevalent at the same time, and reaching forward into wider societal and political repercussions. In short, we can integrate the 'One Health' approach to where these diseases come from with the 'people's science' practice of responding to them.[36]

The policies and practices needed range far beyond the scope of this book, and the pathogen and the pandemy move faster than the publishing calendar, so any details suggested here would be out of date by the time they are in print. The pandemic needs biomedicine and NPIs; the pandemy needs much more. Emancipatory public health begins with a conversation on this whole-of-society, whole-planet, 'One Health', democratic, and participatory agenda. The starting point is not the content of the policies but the process for getting to them. Those who are most vulnerable and most excluded will have some of the most important things to say. This means dismantling the 'war on disease' mindset and its politics, assembled over the last two centuries. If we do this, Covid-19 may yet be the emancipatory catastrophe we need.

Notes

Chapter 1 Following the Science, Following the Script

1 See, among others: Cox 2020; Nie et al. 2016.
2 Osterholm 2005, p. 72; 2020 at 26.00.
3 The scale is reproduced and critiqued in Caduff 2015, pp. 174–5.
4 I discuss this in chapter 5. This definition was for influenza but it transfers readily to Covid-19.
5 A similar form of words was used by the WHO's Bruce Aylward (see Aylward 2020).
6 Murray 2020 at 10.01. A closer parallel might be election forecasting while the candidates are breaking the rules and disrupting the process.
7 Margaret Chan, 'World Now at the Start of 2009 Influenza Pandemic', statement to the press, 11 June 2009.
8 See Kay and King 2020 for an exploration of this issue.
9 The CDC also asked the public not to buy respirator masks, fearing that there would not be enough for health workers.
10 Latour 2017, p. 117.
11 Krieger 2011, p. viii.
12 Quammen 2012, p. 515.
13 Peter Sands is a rare economist who recognizes this (see Sands et al. 2016).

14 Krieger 2011, p. 43; Stefanou-Konidaris 2020.
15 Hanna and Kleinman 2013; Krieger 2011.
16 Larson 2020, p. xxvii.
17 Richards 2016, p. 145.
18 In this book, I am going to keep a respectful distance from the writings of Michel Foucault, but I must acknowledge his insight that the disciplinary powers of the modern state were constructed around apparatuses of excluding, confining, and surveilling communicable diseases. The difficulty of bringing Foucault into such a discussion is that to do justice to his thought and engaging with the literature requires more space than is available.
19 Article 22 of the International Covenant on Civil and Political Rights guarantees freedom of association but carves out exemptions for public health.
20 This refers to the title of Lisa Pisani's 2008 book.

Chapter 2 The Rage of Numbers: Cholera

1 Gradmann 2013, p. 73.
2 Clausewitz 1968.
3 Tilly 1990.
4 Zinsser 1935, p. 153.
5 Zinsser 1935, p. vii. The bacterium responsible for epidemic typhus is named *Rickettsia prowazekii* in honour of its discoverers, the pathologist H.T. Ricketts and his colleague Stan Prowazek, who both contracted typhus and died during their research. Microbiologists in the heroic age of medical research were truly brave and routinely experimented on themselves, sometimes with fatal consequences. See Altman 1987.
6 Smith 1943, p. 205.
7 Cohen 2011.
8 De 1959.
9 Wills 1996, p. 122.
10 Feachem 1982.
11 Peters 1885, p. 3.
12 Arnold 1993, pp. 169–70.
13 Arnold 1993, pp. 168–9.
14 McDonald 1951, pp. 26–8.
15 Peters 1885, p. 10.
16 Henze 2011.

17 Henze 2011, p. 16.
18 Peters 1885, p. 12.
19 Kraikovski 2013; McGrew 1960.
20 Henze 2011, p. 16.
21 Cohn 2010; Slack 1992, p. 15. Note, however, the distinction between what is false and what is unscientific. Astrological theories made precise mathematical predictions and were falsifiable.
22 Pullan 1992, p. 109.
23 Defoe 1722.
24 Ross 2015, p. 11.
25 Evans 1992, p. 164.
26 Quoted in Ross 2015, p. 95.
27 Quoted in Ross 2015, pp. 95–6.
28 Ross 2015, p. 245.
29 Bellinger 2015, p. 218.
30 Bellinger 2015, p. 221.
31 Frevert 2009; Hagemann 1997.
32 Beaney 2009.
33 Pinkard 2000, p. 659.
34 Bronfen 1992.
35 Bellinger 2015.
36 Clausewitz 1968, pp. 101 and 119. There are variant translations, including 'policy' for 'politics' and 'intermixed with other means'. The exact phrase was actually written by Marie (see Bellinger 2015, p. 197).
37 Clausewitz 1968, p. 103.
38 Rothfels 1943, p. 100.
39 Clausewitz 1968, p. 140.
40 Clausewitz 1968, p. 280.
41 Arnold 1993, p. 172.
42 Krieger 2011, p. 77.
43 Gibbon 1782, p. 341.
44 Ackerknecht 2009; see also Hamlin 2009.
45 Ackerknecht 2009, p. 8.
46 Douglas 1966.
47 Wootton 2006.
48 Bernoulli 2004.
49 Colombo and Diamanti 2015.
50 Wootton 2006, p. 157.
51 Delaporte 1986, pp. 11, 78, 139–40.
52 Ackerknecht 2009.

53 Cohn 2017; Delaporte 1986; Evans 1992.
54 Delaporte 1986, p. 60.
55 Cohn 2017.
56 Engels 1892.
57 Cohn 2017, p. 177.
58 Azar 1997; Eisenberg 1986; Virchow 1985.
59 Azar 1997, p. 67.
60 There's a much-recounted tale that Bismarck was so incensed that he challenged Virchow to a duel, inviting him to choose his weapons in accord with custom. The story goes that Virchow received the letter in his laboratory and responded by holding up two apparently identical sausages, one of which was infected with potentially deadly *Trichinella spiralis* roundworm and the other which wasn't. 'Let Bismarck select one and eat it and I will eat the other.' It is, sadly, a myth. *Skulls in the Stars* 2014; Walter and Scott 2017.
61 Cohn 2017, p. 176.
62 Senior Curate of St Luke's 1854, p. 1.
63 Johnson 2006.
64 Wootton 2006, p. 198.
65 Johnson 2006, pp. 174–5.
66 Senior Curate of St Luke's 1854, p. 14.
67 Johnson 2006, p. 211.
68 Ferguson 2011.
69 McDonald 1951, p. 28.
70 Hardy 1993; Maglen 2002; McDonald 1951.
71 Baldwin 1999, p. 534.
72 Watts 1997, pp. 204–7.
73 McClenna 1885.
74 De Waal 2017, pp. 41–3; Mayhew 2014.
75 Dyson 1991. Cholera mortality was often so high that Dyson separately calculates excess death rates with and without cholera.
76 Watts 2001, pp. 347–51.
77 Watts 1997, p. 208.
78 Arnold 1993, p. 161.
79 Peters 1994, p. 302.
80 Zylberman 2007.
81 Velmet 2020.
82 Keller 2006.
83 Pacini was only properly recognized in 1965 when the bacillus was officially renamed *Vibrio cholerae Pacini 1854*.

84 Lippi and Gutozzo 2014, p. 193.
85 Fellow of the Royal Society, Fellow of the Royal Society of Edinburgh, Fellow of the Royal College of Surgeons, Fellow of the Royal College of Physicians, Knight Commander of the Star of India, Master of Law. A Baronet is a heritable knighthood that does not elevate the individual to the House of Lords.
86 Watts 2001, p. 337.
87 Watts 2001, p. 334.
88 Watts 1997, p. 204. They applied similar scepticism to microbial theories of the plague.
89 Altman 1987, p. 23.
90 Morabia 2007; Oppenheimer and Susser 2007.
91 Quoted in Morabia 2007, p. 1235.
92 Evans 1995, pp. 239–40.
93 Cohen 2011, p. 20.
94 Quoted in Gradmann 2013, p. 71.
95 Smallman-Raynor and Cliff 2004, p. 456.
96 Nie 1996.
97 Fuks 2020, pp. 56–7; see also Burnside 1983.
98 Sydenham's observations on disease were derived from his practice among the poor, after he fell from favour after the Restoration of King Charles II in 1660.
99 Quoted in Gradmann 2013, p. 74.
100 Quoted in Gradmann 2013, p. 74.
101 Arnold 1993, p. 164.
102 Henze 2011.
103 Peters 1994, p. 303.
104 Evans 1995, pp. 285–6.
105 Twain 1923, p. 186.
106 Evans 1995, pp. 266–7.
107 Markel 1995, p. 454.
108 This draws heavily on the definitive account by Richard Evans (1995).
109 Evans 1995, pp. 312–13.
110 Altman 1987.
111 Quoted in Altman 1987, p. 25.
112 Evans (1995, pp. 497–8) suggests that Koch's laboratory assistants, who provided the samples, suspected the purpose of the request and mercifully diluted the solutions. An identical experiment was undertaken by his disciple Rudolf Emmerich 10 days later, which he began on a stage in front of an audience of

over a hundred people. Emmerich also fell sick and survived. Pettenkofer finally fulfilled his death wish with a pistol to his temple in 1901.

Chapter 3 Metamorphosis: Influenza

1 Stach 2013, p. 262. The original German is: 'Als Thema der Habsburgermonarchie im Fieber versinken und als Bürger einer tschechischen Demokratie wieder aufwachen: Das war beängstigend, aber auch seltsam.' The translation by Shelley Frisch is, 'certainly eerie, though a bit comical as well'. The translation 'scary and strange' is from 'When Kafka Got the Spanish Flu', 13 April 2020, https://www.web24. news/u/2020/04/when-kafka-got-the-spanish-flu.html; original German version: Drbyos, 'Als Kafka die spanische Grippe bekam', Nach Welt, 12 April 2020, https://nach-welt.com/actionszenen-aus-der-weltliteratur-franz-kafka/.

2 The German *ungeheures Ungeziefer* literally translates as 'monstrous vermin'.

3 Stach 2013, p. 253.

4 Stach 2013, p. 254.

5 Spinney 2017, pp. 166–70.

6 Outka 2019, p. 3.

7 Angell 1910.

8 The Latin word 'virus' meant poisonous liquid. In the early bacteriological age, the term 'filterable virus' was used, 'which meant in effect disease-stuff of unknown composition that could not be separated by filtration from the liquids it was found in' (see Smith 1943, p. 78).

9 A few critics questioned the wisdom of reducing the concept of war to its weapons. After World War I, the epidemiologist and racial theorist Francis Crookshank gave the hypothetical scenario of 'an ingenious police surgeon' who had ascertained the cause of death in a murder case to be a bullet. 'Shortly after he went abroad to a war, and, honestly believing that war is but murder on a large scale, he investigated the appearances of many bodies; again finding bullets, he declared that bullets are the cause of war, as of murder' (Crookshank 1919–20, p. 178). Crookshank elaborates the analogy in amusing ways. For example, noting that some casualties are caused by poison gas, the surgeon concludes that there are in fact two parallel wars.

It is unfortunate that Crookshank's racist theories obscured his other insights.

10 Mehra 2009.

11 Ackerknecht 2009; Krieger 2011, pp. 70–1.

12 Chaves-Carballo 2005.

13 This was probably deliberate, though the disappearance of Lazear's personal diary means that there has been speculation that it was accidental, or an impromptu infection after the young doctor was criticized for not experimenting on himself first. See Mehra 2009. Agramonte, who was assumed to have immunity to yellow fever from exposure during childhood, wasn't an experimental subject.

14 Altman 1987, pp. 143–4, 157–8.

15 Mehra 2009, p. 328.

16 Chaves-Carballo 2013.

17 Stern 2006, p. 46.

18 Smallman-Raynor and Cliff 2004, p. 417. Cholera travelled with the French troops embarking in Marseilles and Toulon, a rare case of it moving from west to east (Evans 1992, p. 161).

19 Seaman 2018, p. 93.

20 Sartin 1993.

21 Zinsser 1935.

22 Morens and Taubenberger 2011; Osterholm and Olshaker 2017, p. 262.

23 CDC 2019.

24 Caduff 2015, p. 99.

25 Morens and Taubenberger 2010.

26 The similarities and differences between influenza and Covid-19 will be explored in chapter 6.

27 If we use the virological definition of pandemic status – a new strain – it's possible that there were pandemics of less virulent strains that passed unnoticed because they didn't kill many people.

28 Morner and Garenne 2000. The data do not allow us to tell whether the gender disparity was due to greater male susceptibility to the disease or the greater exposure of men to infection because they were soldiers. Morner and Garenne link the sex specificity to tuberculosis.

29 Osler 1914.

30 Smallman-Raynor and Cliff 2004, p. 35.

31 Zinsser 1935, pp. 297–9.

32 Mullet 1918, p. 41.
33 E.g. Barry 2005; Crosby 1989.
34 Ewald 1994, p. 110, emphasis added.
35 Ewald 1994 , pp. 67–86.
36 Ewald 2002, pp. 111–12.
37 Byerly 2005, p. 94.
38 Watterson and Kamradt-Scott 2016.
39 Erkoreka 2009, p. 193.
40 Erkoreka 2009, p. 191.
41 Oxford 2001.
42 Cited in Erkoreka 2009, p. 191.
43 Oxford and Gill 2019, p. 2010.
44 Bauer and Vögele 2013.
45 German Office of Sanitation 2013.
46 Byerly 2005, p. 97.
47 Burnet and Clark 1942; Humphries 2014.
48 Barry 2004.
49 Barry 2004.
50 Cf. Beck 2016.
51 Barry 2005, pp. 185–93.
52 Grist 1979, pp. 1632–3.
53 Cited in Kent 2013, p. 103.
54 Barry 2005, p. 171.
55 Byerly 2005, p. 99.
56 Kent 2013, p. 15
57 Wever and van Bergen 2014, p. 544.
58 Barry 2005, p. 9.
59 Barry 2005, p. 343.
60 Eyler 2010.
61 Quoted in Eyler 2010, p. 35.
62 Bruno Latour makes this point in the context of climate change, using Tolstoy's account of Marshal Kutuzov's acceptance of the predetermined course of battle against Napoleon, and the inversion of active agent and inactive object (Latour 2017, pp. 50–1 and 72–4).
63 Byerly 2005, p. 100.
64 Barry 2005, p. 306.
65 Byerly 2005, p. 103.
66 Barry, quoted in Coll 2020.
67 Barry 2005, p. 342.
68 Rosner 2010.

69 Barry and Dickerson 2020.
70 Markel et al. 2007, p. 652.
71 Markel et al. 2007, p. 647.
72 Markel et al. 2007, p. 652.
73 Cited in Tomes 2010, p. 48.
74 A study of 43 cities: Markel et al. 2007. A study of 17 cities: Hatchett et al. 2007.
75 Hatchett et al. 2007.
76 *Gunnison Times*, n.d. 'Gunnison and the Great Influenza', https://www.gunnisontimes.com/content/gunnison-and-great-influenza-0; Markel et al. 2006, p. 1963.
77 Tomes 2010, p. 60.
78 Tomes 2010, p. 59.
79 Bristow 2020; Lipton and Steinhauer 2020.
80 Inglesby et al. 2006, p. 367.
81 Inglesby et al. 2006, pp. 366–7.
82 Lipton and Steinhauer 2020.
83 Phillips 1990.
84 Edgar and Sapire 1999, p. 7.
85 Ranger 1992, p. 245.
86 Ranger 1992, p. 264.
87 Cheng and Leung 2007.
88 Segal 2020.
89 Quoted in Killingray 2003, p. 32.
90 Barry 2020.
91 Outka 2019.
92 Huizinga 1924, p. 1. (The original Dutch language edition was published in 1919.)
93 Thompson 1921, p. 565.
94 Thompson 1921, p. 566.
95 Ziegler 1969, p. 288.
96 McNeill 1977.
97 Crosby 1989. (The first edition was published in 1976 with the title *Epidemic and Peace, 1918*.)
98 Barry 2020 at 7.30.
99 Edgar and Sapire 1999, p. xxii. See also Vaughan 1991, p. 102, on the challenge facing the historian trying to hear the voices of ordinary Africans, especially those categorized as 'mad', in the colonial era.
100 Kolko 1994, p. 8.
101 Ferguson 1999, p. 462, emphasis in original.

102 Zinsser 1935, p. 152.
103 Phillips 2004.
104 Bristow 2017, p. 11.
105 Watterson and Scott 2016.
106 Spellberg and Taylor-Blake 2013.
107 Jordan et al. 2019.
108 Taubenberger et al. 1997.
109 Reid et al. 1999; Reid et al. 2000.
110 Jordan et al. 2019.
111 Tumpey et al. 2005, p. 79.
112 Ewald 2002, p. 25.
113 Morens et al. 2009, p. 228.
114 Spinney 2017, pp. 290–3.
115 Crosby 1989.
116 Blickle 2020.
117 Isherwoood 2008, p. 181.
118 Barry 2020, at 9.55.
119 Bristow 2017.
120 Outka 2019.
121 Onion 2020.
122 Outka 2019, pp. 142–5.
123 Barry 2005, pp. 382–8.
124 See MacMillan 2003. MacMillan does not attribute Wilson's incapacitation to any particular cause.
125 Hoover 2013, pp. 118–19.
126 Hoover 2013, p. 119.
127 Holohan 2017, p. 118.
128 Tuchman 1979, p. 105. See Cohn 2010 for vernacular literature and practical manuals.
129 Cantor 2002, p. 213. Intriguingly, Cantor also makes the point that the impact of the plague was to be seen most clearly in the prominent individuals whom it felled, for example Princess Joan Plantaganet (p. 81).
130 Ziegler 1969, p. 288.
131 Ziegler 1969, p. 288.

Chapter 4 Who, Whom: HIV/AIDS

1 De Waal 2006, pp. 117–19; Isabirye 2008.
2 Anderson 2003.
3 Pepin 2011, pp. 36–9.

4 Daughton 2011, p. 515.

5 This draws on Pisani 2008.

6 Watts et al. 2010.

7 For a general discussion of this see Pisani 2008, esp. pp. 128–42; for key epidemiological studies, see Alary and Lowndes 2004; Morris and Kretzschmar 1997; Piot et al. 1987.

8 Andrews and Rowland-Jones 2017.

9 Hutchinson 2003, p. 50.

10 For an accessible account of the viral origins of HIV, see Crawford 2013.

11 Sauter and Kirchhoff 2019.

12 Crawford 2013, pp. 103–4; Quammen 2012, pp. 468–77.

13 Sauter and Kirchhoff 2019.

14 Crawford 2013, p. 82; Tompa 2017.

15 African governments resented the implication that Africa was the source of AIDS, that it was a disease of homosexuals, and that they were facing unrecognized epidemics. The Kenyan government seized all copies of an issue of the *New York Times* with an article on AIDS in Africa in 1985.

16 Shilts 1987.

17 Wald 2008, pp. 215–16. According to some reports, Dugas was also patient 'O' for 'outside California', not '0' for 'zero' (see Racaniello 2016).

18 Worobey et al. 2016.

19 Curtis 1992.

20 Hooper 1999.

21 Crawford 2013, pp. 133–49.

22 Those wanting to rubbish Hooper's book didn't review it. For a reflective review, see Lucas 2000.

23 Crawford 2013, pp. 45–6.

24 Crawford 2013, pp. 46–7; Pepin 2011, pp. 170–4.

25 Gisselquist et al. 2003.

26 Pepin 2011.

27 Velmet 2020, esp. pp. 6–20.

28 Pepin 2011, pp. 120–4.

29 Velmet 2020, pp. 103–4.

30 Quoted in Pepin 2011, p. 164.

31 De Cock 2012.

32 White 1990.

33 Alary and Lowndes 2004; Piot et al. 1987.

34 Vaughan 1991, pp. 129–54.

35 Pepin 2011, pp. 162–3; Vaughan 1991, pp. 138–40.
36 Faria et al. 2015.
37 Yebra et al. 2015.
38 Wilkinson et al. 2015.
39 Pepin 2011, p. 196.
40 Pepin 2011, pp. 200–5.
41 Barnett and Blaikie 1992; Obbo 1993.
42 Shoumatoff 1988.
43 Kaplan 1994.
44 Hooper 1999, pp. 42–9; Ondoga ori Amaza 1998, pp. 148–9; UNAIDS 1998; Yeager et al. 2000.
45 Allen 2006; de Waal et al. 2009.
46 Paxton 2014; Spiegel 2004; Whiteside et al. 2006.
47 Foss et al. 2008; Supervie et al. 2010.
48 African Rights 2004.
49 For the clearest exposition of this, see Pisani 2008. An example is that outside eastern and southern Africa, instead of targeting HIV interventions at groups such as sex workers and their clients, AIDS education was directed at the whole population – a poor use of scarce money and time.
50 Barnett and Whiteside 2002; Whiteside 2008.
51 For this debate, see Caldwell et al. 1989; Tamale 2011.
52 Epprecht 2013.
53 De Waal et al. 2009, pp. 108–11; Spiegel 2004.
54 Shell 1999.
55 Campbell 2003.
56 Watts et al. 2010.
57 Pisani 2008, p. 173.
58 Kenyon and Buyze 2015.
59 Raguin et al. 2011; Smith et al. 2009; Strathdee and Stockman 2010; Van Griensven 2007. On the controversy over iatrogenic infection, see Gisselquist et al. 2003.
60 United States Department of Health and Human Resources, Press Conference Secretary Margaret Heckler, 23 April 1984, transcript at https://quod.lib.umich.edu/c/cohenaids/5571095.0 488.004?rgn=main;view=fulltext .
61 In 1989, an HIV-positive man was prevented from entering the United States to attend a conference in San Francisco, after which there was a massive boycott of the sixth international HIV/AIDS conference in that city the following year. The entry ban for HIV-positive people was formalized in 1991 and

lifted only in 2010, after which San Francisco was chosen to host the July 2020 international HIV/AIDS conference – postponed because of Covid-19.

62 Chan 2015; Epstein 1996.
63 Mann et al. 1994; Piot 2012.
64 Machel 1975, pp. 48 and 56.
65 Tumushabe 2005, p. 8.
66 De Waal 2006, pp. 106–7; UNECA 2001.
67 De Waal 2006, p. 107.
68 De Waal 2006, pp. 98–9.
69 Tumushabe 2005, p. 12.
70 Dowden 2009, pp. 321–53.
71 Buse et al. 2008.
72 Whiteside et al. 2003.
73 Achmat 2004; Heywood 2005; Mbali 2005.
74 Chan 2015; Pisani 2008.
75 Davis and Feshbach 1980.
76 Eberstadt 2006 (originally published 1981).
77 Eberstadt 1988 (essays published during 1981–8.)
78 Esty et al. 1995.
79 Elbe 2009, pp. 9–10.
80 Kaldor 2012.
81 CIA 1987.
82 The White House, Office of Science and Technology, 'Addressing the Threat of Emerging Infectious Diseases', and Office of the Vice President, 'Vice President Announces Policy on Infectious Diseases: New presidential policy calls for coordinated approach to global issue', 12 July 1996, https://fas.org/irp/offdocs/pdd_ntsc7.htm.
83 National Intelligence Council 2000.
84 National Intelligence Council 2002; UN Theme Group on HIV/AIDS and China 2002.
85 Blacker and Zaba 1997.
86 I calculated the figures for seven African and four non-African countries (de Waal 2006, pp. 4–5).
87 De Waal 2003; Elbe 2003; Fourie and Schönteich 2001; Garrett 2005; McPherson et al. 2000; Neilson 2005; Pharoah 2004; Schönteich 2000; Whiteside and de Waal 2003.
88 Commission on HIV/AIDS and Governance in Africa 2008; de Waal et al. 2009; Joint Learning Initiative on Children and HIV/AIDS 2009; see also de Waal 2006; 2010.

89 There is a big literature on fragile states and on the critique of the paradigm.
90 Haacker 2004; World Bank 1999.
91 I did this search on 13 December 2020. The first 15 were all either icons or pictures; of the next 15, 11 were so; thereafter it was about half.
92 North 1991, p. 97.
93 De Waal 2015.
94 Piot 2013, p. 376.
95 Sontag 1988, p. 183.
96 De Waal et al. 2009, p. 75.
97 Pisani 2008, p. 51.
98 Pisani 2008, pp. 307 and 9.
99 Petro 2015.
100 Hamlin 2009, commenting on Ackerknecht 2009, uses the same comparison.

Chapter 5 Imagined Unknowns: Pandemic X

1 Calisher et al. 2006, p. 539.
2 Piot 2012; Preston 1994.
3 Another fictionalized version took the form of a scenario of an outbreak of airborne Ebola in an African refugee camp infecting hundreds of refugees and a small number of international aid workers who brought the disease to the United States. This scenario was presented at the opening session of the 1989 conference of the American Society for Tropical Medicine and Hygiene (Henig 1994, pp. 217–19).
4 Garrett 1994.
5 Quammen 2012, p. 42.
6 Henig 1994, p. 36
7 For the full list of criteria, see WHO 2018, p. 12.
8 Wald 2008.
9 Wald 2008, p. 2.
10 Players win the board game *Pandemic* when they collaboratively find cures for four epidemic diseases. The cover design for the game includes the figures of four protagonists (scientist, army doctor, operations director and contingency planner), a helicopter, and a fighter jet, though the fighter plane actually has no role in the game.
11 Preston 1994, pp. 93–5.

12 Lederberg et al. Oaks 1992.
13 Cueto et al. 2019, pp. 245–6.
14 WHO 1998, pp. 541 and 542 (it is a reprint of the original 1994 meeting memo).
15 Charon 2008.
16 Semino et al. 2018.
17 Douglas 1986.
18 Davies et al. 2015, pp. 22–4.
19 Fidler 1999.
20 Fidler 2003, p. 487.
21 Butler 1994; Garrett 2000, pp. 15–49.
22 Garrett 2000, p. 48.
23 Bartels et al. 2010.
24 Chigudu 2020.
25 Davies et al. 2015, p. 32.
26 WHO 1997.
27 Chan 2002.
28 Snacken et al. 1999.
29 Vandegrift et al. 2010.
30 Davis 2005.
31 Sands et al. 2016.
32 Johns Hopkins 2001; O'Toole et al. 2002.
33 Rumsfeld 2002.
34 Musk 2020.
35 FBI 2010.
36 Hayden 2011, p. 152.
37 President of the United States 2010, pp. 48–9.
38 Caduff 2015, p. 176.
39 Bush 2005.
40 Preston 1994, pp. 149–50.
41 Preston 1994, p. 92.
42 Rhodes 1986, pp. 664–5.
43 Perrow 1984.
44 Schlosser 2013, p. 464.
45 *Bulletin of the Atomic Scientists*, website, https://thebulletin.org/about-us/#.
46 Furmanski 2014.
47 Rozo and Gronvall 2015; Wertheim 2010.
48 E.g. Rozo and Gronvall 2015.
49 Klotz 2019.
50 Imai et al. 2012; University of Wisconsin-Madison 2012.

51 Furmanski 2015; Piper 2020.
52 See Michael Osterholm's comments in Schnirring 2017.
53 Lakoff 2017, p. 138.
54 Schnirring 2017.
55 Racaniello 2020.
56 For examples see Piot 2012, p. 61 and Preston 1994, pp. 157–9.
57 Quammen 2012, pp. 199–202 (SARS in China) and pp. 352–5 (Marburg in Uganda).
58 CNN 2020, at 9.01.
59 Kleinman and Watson 2005, p. 1.
60 Huang 2004, p. 119.
61 Huang 2004, p. 118,
62 Kamradt-Scott 2015, p. 97.
63 The WHO representative in Beijing, Henk Bekedam, also criticized China's unwillingness to cooperate fully with the WHO and went on to denounce the failings of the Chinese health system.
64 Fidler 2003.
65 Davies et al. 2015, pp. 44–5, 49–50, and 56.
66 Kaufman 2005. Note that UNAIDS and the US National Intelligence Council both published reports highly critical of China's HIV/AIDS policies in 2002. In 2003, China also changed its AIDS policies.
67 Pomfret 2003.
68 Yang 2020.
69 Zhang 2005, p. 157.
70 Lee and McKibbin 2004, p. 103.
71 Peckham 2016; Xiang 2020.
72 Fidler 2020.
73 Saich 2005.
74 Saich 2020.
75 Lynteris 2016, emphasis in the original.
76 Atem 2017, p. 127.
77 Piot 2012, pp. 56–7.
78 Davies et al. 2015, p. 104.
79 Martin and Krauss 2009.
80 Martin and Krauss 2009.
81 *National Hog Farmer* 2009.
82 WHO 2015.
83 Kupferschmidt 2015.
84 The same issue arises with famine early warning.

85 CDC n.d.
86 Cohen 2009; Doshi 2011; Kelly 2011.
87 Koblenz 2009; Normile 2005.
88 Davis 2005.
89 Kamradt-Scott 2015, p. 164.
90 Lakoff 2017, pp. 141–51. Compare the National Intelligence Council reports of 2000, 2002, and 2008 to see this shift for HIV/AIDS.
91 Piot 2012, p. 50.
92 Piot 2012, p. 51.
93 De Waal 2006, pp. 24–5; Desmond et al. 2004.
94 Piot 2012, p. 69.
95 Meltzer et al. 2014; see also Meltzer et al. 2016.
96 Cui 2019.
97 Brooks 2016.
98 Walsh and Johnson 2018, p. 218.
99 Walsh and Johnson 2018, p. 303.
100 De Waal 2014; see also Benton 2017.
101 Benton 2017.
102 Farmer 2003.
103 Farmer 2014.
104 This was an important and often neglected point: there was a collapse of child health services, obstetrics, and vaccination. During the epidemic in Sierra Leone, there were 3,956 deaths from Ebola and an estimated 2,819 additional malaria deaths because medical services were dealing only with Ebola (see Ribacke et al. 2016).
105 Walsh and Johnson 2018, p. 276. Another example was a leading health agency discouraging others with less experience from opening programmes because they could not guarantee the highest standards of care.
106 Walsh and Johnson 2018, p. 121.
107 Walsh and Johnson 2018, pp. 124 and 333.
108 Akanni 2014.
109 Parker et al. 2019.
110 Parker et al. 2019, p. 446.
111 Benton 2017, p. 38.
112 Sinead and Johnson 2018, p. 342.
113 Farmer 2014.
114 Sinead and Johnson 2018, p. 303.
115 Richards 2016, pp. 3–9.

116 Richards 2016, pp. 18 and 51–2.
117 Cueto et al. 2019, pp. 324–6; Kirchoff 2016; Moon et al. 2015.
118 Parker et al. 2019, p. 441.
119 Bar-Yam 2016.
120 Kirchhoff 2016, p. 3.
121 Richards 2016, p. 145.

Chapter 6 Emancipatory Catastrophe? Covid-19

1 GPMB 2019, p. 6. By comparison, Covid-19 killed 1.65 million people in its first year and wiped 5 per cent off global GDP – i.e. we were *over*-warned.
2 Respectively, former Director General of the WHO and Secretary General of the International Federation of Red Cross and Red Crescent Societies.
3 GPMB 2020, p. 3.
4 Johns Hopkins Center for Health Security 2019.
5 CSIS Commission on Strengthening America's Health Security 2019.
6 GPMB 2020, p. 6.
7 GPMB 2019, p. 24.
8 Caduff 2020.
9 For a summary, see XinhuaNet 2020.
10 Hana et al. 2020.
11 Kuo 2016.
12 *Asahi Shimbun*, 'Emperor Marks War Anniversary with Call to Rally on COVID-19', 15 August 2020.
13 See Caduff 2020 for a vigorous critique of the standard response.
14 See Scoones 2020 for a timely incisive dissection of this; also Scoones et al. 2017.
15 Ferguson et al. 2020, p. 3. See also Murray 2020 at 15.45: 'Our models may be wrong, but at least we can have something out there to say, here's how we got to those dates [for reopening states].'
16 Bank 2020.
17 Davidson and Rees-Mogg 1999, p. i.
18 Davidson and Rees-Mogg 1999, p. 18.
19 Rand 1999, p. 279. The line quoted shows a rudimentary misunderstanding of how life expectancy is calculated.
20 Peikoff 1991, p. 342.
21 Joyner 2018.

22 Gomel 2000, pp. 422–3.
23 De Waal 2015.
24 Nagel 1974.
25 Nagel 1974, p. 447.
26 Nagel 1974, p. 445.
27 Caduff 2015, pp. 88 and 99.
28 The words attributed to Pasteur are, 'Gentlemen, it is the microbes who will have the last word.'
29 Calisher et al. 2006.
30 Plowright et al. 2011; Quammen 2012, pp. 366–9.
31 Bar-On et al. 2018; Osane 2018.
32 Morens and Fauci 2020, p. 1089.
33 Council on Foreign Relations 2020; GPMB 2020.
34 Caduff 2015, p. 34.
35 Beck 2016, p. 15.
36 See Scoones et al. 2017 for the 'three Ps' approach to this: *process* (the way disease population dynamics work), *pattern* (the spatial spread of disease and the correlation with various factors), and *participation* (understanding disease dynamics from local people's perspectives).

References

Achmat, Zackie, 2004. 'AIDS and Human Rights: A new South African struggle', 2004 John Foster Lecture, 10 November.

Ackerknecht, Edwin H., 2009. 'Anticontagionism between 1821 and 1867: The Fielding H. Garrison Lecture', *International Journal of Epidemiology*, 38: 7-21 (originally published 1948).

African Rights, 2004, *Rwanda: Broken Bodies, Torn Spirits: Living with genocide, rape and HIV/ AIDS*. Kigali: African Rights.

Akanni, Tooni, 2014. 'Confronting Ebola in Liberia: The gendered realities', *Open Democracy*, 20 October, https://www.opendemocracy.net/en/5050/confronting-ebola-in-liberia-gendered-realities-0/

Alary, Michel, and Catherine Lowndes, 2004. 'The Central Role of Clients of Female Sex Workers in the Dynamics of Heterosexual HIV Transmission in sub-Saharan Africa', *AIDS*, 18.6: 945–7.

Allen, Tim, 2006. 'AIDS and Evidence: Interrogating some Ugandan myths', *Journal of Biosocial Science*, 38.1: 7–28.

Altman, Lawrence, 1987. *Who Goes First? The story of*

self-experimentation in medicine. Berkeley: University of California Press.

Anderson, Roy, 2003. 'Keynote Address'. *Report of the Scientific Meeting on the Empirical Evidence for the Demographic and Socio-economic Impact of AIDS*, Durban, 26–8 March.

Andrews, Sophie, and Sarah Rowland-Jones, 2017. 'Recent Advances in Understanding HIV Evolution', *F1000Research*, 6: 597. doi:10.12688/f1000research.10876.1

Angell, Norman, 1910. *The Great Illusion: A study of the relation of military power to national advantage*. New York: G.B. Putnam.

Arnold, David, 1993. *Colonizing the Body: State medicine and epidemic disease in nineteenth-century India*. Berkeley: University of California Press.

Atem, Atem Yaak, 2017. *Jungle Chronicles and Other Writings: Recollections of a South Sudanese*. Perth: Africa World Books.

Aylward, Bruce, 2020. 'We Have to Learn to Respect the Virus – and Learn as the Disease Evolves', *New Scientist*, 16 March. https://www.newscientist.com/article/2237493-we-have-to-respect-the-coronavirus-and-learn-as-the-disease-evolves/

Azar, Henry, 1997. 'Rudolf Virchow, Not Just a Pathologist: A re-examination of the report on the typhus epidemic in Upper Silesia', *Annals of Diagnostic Pathology*, 1.1: 65–71.

Baldwin, Peter, 1999. *Contagion and the State in Europe, 1830–1930*. New York: Cambridge University Press.

Bank, Leslie, 2020. 'Beyond a Bio-medical Fix – The value of "people's science"', *University World News, Africa Edition*, 30 April. https://www.universityworldnews.com/post.php?story=20200429151310413

Barnett, Tony, and Piers Blaikie, 1992. *AIDS in Africa: Its present and future impact*. London: Guilford Press.

Barnett, Tony, and Alan Whiteside, 2002. *AIDS in the Twenty-First Century: Disease and globalization*. London: Palgrave Macmillan.

Bar-On, Yinon M., Rob Phillips, and Ron Milo, 2018. 'The Biomass Distribution on Earth', *Proceedings of the National Academy of Sciences*, 115.25: 6506–11.

Barry, Dan, and Caitlin Dickerson, 2020, 'The Killer Flu of 1918: A Philadelphia story', *New York Times*, 4 April. https://www.nytimes.com/2020/04/04/us/coronavirus-spanish-flu-philadelphia-pennsylvania.html

Barry, John, 2004. 'The Site of Origin of the 1918 Influenza Pandemic and Its Public Health Implications', *Journal of Translational Medicine* 2.1: 3. doi: 10.1186/1479-5876-2-3

Barry, John, 2005. *The Great Influenza: The story of the greatest pandemic in history.* New York: Penguin.

Barry, John, 2020. 'Coronavirus Crisis Update: John Barry, eminent pandemic historian – "Tell the truth"', Center for Strategic and International Studies podcast, *Take as Directed*, 15 May. https://www.csis.org/podcasts/take-directed-coronavirus-crisis-update

Bartels, Susan, P. Gregg Greenough, M. Tamar, and Michael VanRooyen, 2010. 'Investigation of a Cholera Outbreak in Ethiopia's Oromiya Region', *Disaster Medicine and Public Health Preparedness*, 4.4: 312–17.

Bar-Yam, Yaneer, 2016. 'How Community Response Stopped Ebola', *New England Complex Systems Institute*, 11 July. https://necsi.edu/how-community-response-stopped-ebola

Bauer, Frieder, and Jörg Vögele, 2013. 'Die "Spanische Grippe" in der Deutschen Armee 1918 – Perspektive der Ärzte und Generäle/The "Spanish Flu" in the German Army 1918 – the perspectives of physicians and generals', *Medizinhistorisches Journal* 48.2: 117–52.

Beaney, Tara, 2009. 'Beautiful Death: The nineteenth-century fascination with *Antigone*', *Opticon1826*, 7.

Beck, Ulrich, 2016. *The Metamorphosis of the World: How climate change is transforming our concept of the world.* Cambridge: Polity.

Bellinger, Vanya Efrimova, 2015. *Marie von Clausewitz: The woman behind the making of On War.* Oxford: Oxford University Press.

Benton, Adia, 2017. 'Whose Security? Militarization and securitization during west Africa's Ebola outbreak', in Michiel Hofman and Sokhieng Au (eds), *The Politics of Fear:*

Médecins sans Frontières and the west African Ebola epidemic. Oxford: Oxford University Press.

Bernoulli, Daniel, 2004. 'An Attempt at a New Analysis of the Mortality Caused by Smallpox and of the Advantages of Inoculation to Prevent It' (reviewed by Sally Blower), *Reviews in Medical Virology*, 14: 275–88.

Blacker, John, and Basia Zaba, 1997. 'HIV Prevalence and Lifetime Risk of Dying of AIDS', *Health Transition Review*, 7, Suppl. 2: 45–62.

Blickle, Kristian, 2020. 'Pandemics Change Cities: Municipal spending and voter extremism in Germany, 1918–1933', FRB of New York Staff Report No. 921, May. Available at SSRN: https://ssrn.com/abstract=3592888 or http://dx.doi.org/10.2139/ssrn.3592888

Bristow, Nancy, 2017. *American Pandemic: The lost worlds of the 1918 influenza epidemic.* Oxford: Oxford University Press.

Bristow, Nancy, 2020. 'What the 1918 Flu Pandemic Tells Us about Whether Social Distancing Works', *The Guardian*, 29 April. https://www.theguardian.com/commentisfree/2020/apr/29/us-responses-1918-flu-pandemic-offer-stark-lessons-coronavirus-now

Bronfen, Elisabeth, 1992. *Over Her Dead Body: Femininity, death and the aesthetic.* London: Routledge.

Brooks, Rosa, 2016. *How Everything Became War and the Military Became Everything: Tales from the Pentagon.* New York: Simon & Schuster.

Burnet, F.M., and Ellen Clark, 1942. *Influenza: A survey of the last 50 years in the light of modern work on the virus of epidemic influenza.* Melbourne: Macmillan.

Burnside, John, 1983. 'Medicine and War – A metaphor', *Journal of the American Medical Association*, 249: 2091.

Buse, Kent, Claire Dickinson, and Michel Sidibé, 2008. 'HIV: Know your epidemic, act on its politics', *Journal of the Royal Society of Medicine*, 101.12: 572–3.

Bush, George W., 2005. 'President Outlines Pandemic

Influenza Preparations and Response'. William Natcher Center, National Institutes of Health, Bethesda, Maryland, 1 November. https://georgewbush-whitehouse.archives.gov/news/releases/2005/11/print/20051101-1.html

Butler, Declan, 1994. 'India Ponders the Flaws Exposed by plague', *Nature*, 372: 119.

Byerly, Carol, 2005. *Fever of War: The influenza epidemic in the US Army during World War I*. New York: New York University Press.

Caduff, Carlo, 2015. *The Pandemic Perhaps: Dramatic events in a public culture of danger*. Berkeley: University of California Press.

Caduff, Carlo, 2020. 'What Went Wrong: Corona and the world after the full stop', *Medical Anthropology Quarterly*, July. doi: 10.1111/maq.12599

Caldwell, John, Pat Caldwell, and Pat Quiggin, 1989. 'The Social Context of AIDS in sub-Saharan Africa', *Population and Development Review*, 15.2: 185–234.

Calisher, Charles, James Childs, Hume Field, et al., 2006. 'Bats: Important reservoir hosts of emerging viruses', *Clinical Microbiology Reviews*, 19.3: 531–45.

Campbell, Horace, 2003. *Reclaiming Zimbabwe: The exhaustion of the patriarchal model of liberation*. Claremont: David Phillips.

Cantor, Norman, 2002. *In the Wake of the Plague: The Black Death and the world it made*. New York: Perennial.

CDC, 2019. 'Types of Influenza Viruses', Atlanta: Centers for Disease Control and Prevention. https://www.cdc.gov/flu/about/viruses/types.htm

CDC, n.d. '2009 H1N1 Pandemic (H1N1pdm09 Virus)', Atlanta: Centers for Disease Control and Prevention. https://www.cdc.gov/flu/pandemic-resources/2009-h1n1-pandemic.html

Chan, Jennifer, 2015. *Politics in the Corridor of the Dying: AIDS activism and global health governance*. Baltimore, MD: Johns Hopkins University Press.

Chan, Paul K.S., 2002. 'Outbreak of Avian Influenza A(H5N1)

Virus Infection in Hong Kong in 1997', *Clinical Infectious Diseases*, 34.2: S58–64.

Charon, Rita, 2008. *Narrative Medicine: Honoring the stories of illness.* Oxford: Oxford University Press.

Chaves-Carballo, Enrique, 2005. 'Carlos Finlay and Yellow Fever: Triumph over adversity', *Military Medicine*, 170.10: 881–5.

Chaves-Carballo, Enrique, 2013. 'Clara Maass, Yellow Fever and Human Experimentation', *Military Medicine* 175.5: 557–62.

Cheng, K.F., and P.C. Leung, 2007. 'What Happened in China during the 1918 Influenza Pandemic?', *International Journal of Infectious Diseases*, 11: 360–4.

Chigudu, Simukai, 2020. *The Political Life of an Epidemic: Cholera, crisis and citizenship in Zimbabwe.* Cambridge: Cambridge University Press.

CIA, 1987. 'Sub-Saharan Africa: Implications of the AIDS pandemic', SNIE-70/1-87, Washington, DC. Redacted version made public in 2001, https://www.cia.gov/library/readingroom/docs/DOC_0000579143.pdf

Clausewitz, Carl von, 1968. *On War*, translated by J.J. Graham, edited by F.N. Maude. London: Penguin (originally published 1832).

CNN, 2020. 'Virus Hunters: CNN Chief Medical Correspondent Dr Sanjay Gupta talks to Dr Peter Daszak', 9 March. https://www.cnn.com/audio/podcasts/corona-virus?episodeguid=3ffef0bd75d5a03515b9d490f3614eb1.mp3

Cohen, Ed, 2011. 'The Paradoxical Politics of Viral Containment; Or, how scale undoes us one and all', *Social Text 106*, 29.1: 15–35.

Cohen, Elizabeth, 2009. 'When a Pandemic Isn't a Pandemic', *CNN*, 4 May, http://edition.cnn.com/2009/HEALTH/05/04/swine.flu.pandemic/index.html

Cohn, Samuel K., 2010. *Cultures of Plague: Medical thinking at the end of the Renaissance.* Oxford: Oxford University Press.

Cohn, Samuel K., 2017. 'Cholera Revolts: A class struggle we may not like', *Social History*, 42:2: 162–80.

Coll, Steve, 2020. 'Woodrow Wilson's Case of the Flu, and How Pandemics Change History', *The New Yorker*, 17 April. https://www.newyorker.com/news/daily-comment/woodrow-wilsons-case-of-the-flu-and-how-pandemics-change-history

Colombo, Camilla, and Mirko Diamanti, 2015. 'The Smallpox Vaccine: The dispute between Bernouilli and d'Alembert and the calculus of probabilities' (translated by Kim Williams), *Lettera Matematica*, 2.4: 185–92.

Commission on HIV/AIDS and Governance in Africa, 2008. *Securing our Future, the Report of the Commission on HIV/AIDS and Governance in Africa*. Addis Ababa: UN Economic Commission for Africa.

Council on Foreign Relations, 2020. 'Improving Pandemic Preparedness: Lessons from COVID-19', Independent Task Force Report No. 78, New York: Council on Foreign Relations.

Cox, Patrick, 2020. 'Fires, Orchestras, Parachutes: Some other ways to describe coronavirus – besides war', *The World*, April 28. https://www.pri.org/stories/2020-04-28/fires-orchestras-parachutes-some-other-ways-describe-coronavirus-besides-war

Crawford, Dorothy, 2013. *Virus Hunt: The search for the origins of HIV*. Oxford: Oxford University Press.

Crookshank, Francis G., 1919–20. 'First Principles: And Epidemiology', *Proceedings of the Royal Society of Medicine, Section of Epidemiology and State Medicine*, 13: 159–80.

Crosby, Alfred, 1989. *America's Forgotten Pandemic: The influenza of 1918*. New York: Cambridge University Press.

CSIS Commission on Strengthening America's Health Security, 2019. 'Ending the Cycle of Crisis and Complacency in US Global Health Security'. Washington, DC, CSIS, November.

Cueto, Marcos, Theodore Brown, and Elizabeth Fee, 2019. *The World Health Organization: A history*. Cambridge: Cambridge University Press.

Cui, Shunji, 2019. 'China in the Fight against the Ebola Crisis:

Human security perspectives', in Carolina Hernandez, Eun Mee Kim, Yoichi Mine, and Ren Xiao (eds), *Human Security and Cross-border Cooperation in Asia*. London: Palgrave, pp. 155–80.

Curtis, Tom, 1992. 'The Origin of AIDS', *Rolling Stone*, 626: 54–60.

Daughton, J.P., 2011. 'Behind the Imperial Curtain: International humanitarian efforts and the critique of French colonialism in the interwar years', *French Historical Studies*, 34.3: 503–28.

Davidson, James Dale, and William Rees-Mogg, 1999. *The Sovereign Individual: Mastering the transition to the information age*, London: Touchstone.

Davies, Sara, Adam Kamradt-Scott, and Simon Rushton, 2015. *Disease Diplomacy: International norms and global health security*. Baltimore, MD: Johns Hopkins University Press.

Davis, Christopher, and Murray Feshbach, 1980. 'Rising Soviet Infant Mortality', *INTERCOM*, 8.17: 12–14.

Davis, Mike, 2005. *The Monster at Our Door: The global threat of avian flu*. New York: Henry Holt.

De, Sambhu Nath, 1959. 'Enterotoxicity of Bacteria-free Culture-filtrate of *Vibrio cholerae*', *Nature* 183: 1533–4.

De Cock, Kevin, 2012. 'The Origins of AIDS', *Emerging Infectious Diseases*, 18.7: 1215.

de Waal, Alex, 2003. 'How Will HIV/AIDS Transform African Governance?', *African Affairs*, 102: 1–24.

de Waal, Alex, 2006. *AIDS and Power: Why there is no political crisis – yet*. London: International African Institute and Zed Books.

de Waal, Alex, 2010. 'Reframing Governance, Security and Conflict in the Light of HIV/AIDS', *Social Science and Medicine*, 70.1: 114–20.

de Waal, Alex, 2014. 'Militarizing Global Health', *Boston Review*, 11 November. http://bostonreview.net/world/alex-de-waal-militarizing-global-health-ebola

de Waal, Alex, 2015. *The Real Politics of the Horn of Africa: Money, war and the business of power*. Cambridge: Polity.

de Waal, Alex, 2017. *Mass Starvation: The history and future of famine*. Cambridge: Polity.

de Waal, Alex, Jennifer Klot, and Manjari Mahanjan, 2009. *HIV/AIDS, Security and Conflict: New realities, new responses*. New York: Social Science Research Council and The Hague: Clingendael Institute, HIV/AIDS, Security and Conflict Final Report.

Defoe, Daniel, 1722. *A Journal of the Plague Year*. https://www.gutenberg.org/files/376/376-h/376-h.htm

Delaporte, François, 1986. *Disease and Civilization: The cholera in Paris, 1832* (translated by Arthur Goldhammer). Cambridge, MA: MIT Press.

Desmond, Christopher, John King, Jane Tomlinson, et al., 2004. 'Using an Undertaker's Data to Assess Changing Patterns of Mortality and Their Consequences in Swaziland', *African Journal of AIDS Research*, 3.1: 43–50.

Doshi, Peter, 2011. 'The Elusive Definition of Pandemic Influenza', *Bulletin of the World Health Organization*, 89: 532–8.

Douglas, Mary, 1966. *Purity and Danger: An analysis of the concepts of pollution and taboo*. London: Kegan Paul.

Douglas, Mary, 1986. *How Institutions Think*, Syracuse, NY: Syracuse University Press.

Dowden, Richard, 2009. *Africa: Altered states, ordinary miracles*. London: Portobello.

Dyson, Tim, 1991. 'On the Demography of South Asian Famines: Part I', *Population Studies*, 45.1: 5–25.

Eberstadt, Nick, 1988. *The Poverty of Communism*. New York: Transaction Publishers.

Eberstadt, Nick, 2006. 'The Health Crisis in the USSR', *International Journal of Epidemiology*, 35.6: 1384–94 (originally published 1981).

Edgar, Robert, and Hillary Sapire, 1999. *African Apocalypse: The story of Nontetha Nkwenkwe, a twentieth-century prophet*. Athens, OH: Ohio University Press.

Eisenberg, Leon, 1986. 'Rudolf Virchow: The physician as politician', *Medicine and War*, 2:4: 243–50.

Elbe, Stefan, 2009. *Strategic Implications of HIV/AIDS*. London: International Institute for Security Studies, Adelphi Paper 357.

Engels, Friedrich, 1892. *The Condition of the Working Class in England, Preface to the English Edition*. https://www.marxists.org/archive/marx/works/1892/01/11.htm

Epprecht, Mark, 2013. *Sexuality and Social Justice in Africa: Rethinking homophobia and forging resistance*. London: International African Institute and Zed Books.

Epstein, Steven, 1996. *Impure Science: AIDS, activism and the politics of knowledge*. Berkeley: University of California Press.

Erkoreka, Anton, 2009. 'Origins of the Spanish Influenza Pandemic (1918–1920) and Its Relation to the First World War', *Journal of Molecular and Genetic Medicine*, 3: 190–4.

Esty, Daniel C., Jack A. Goldstone, Ted Robert Gurr, Pamela T. Surko, and Alan N. Unger 1995. *State Failure Task Force Report*. Washington, DC: State Failure Task Force.

Evans, Richard, 1992. 'Epidemics and Revolutions: Cholera in nineteenth-century Europe', in Terence Ranger and Paul Slack (eds), *Epidemics and Ideas: Essays on the historical perception of pestilence*. Cambridge: Cambridge University Press, pp. 149–74.

Evans, Richard, 1995. *Death in Hamburg: Society and politics in the Cholera years*, Second edition. London: Penguin.

Ewald, Paul, 1994. *Evolution of Infectious Disease*. Oxford: Oxford University Press.

Ewald, Paul, 2002. *Plague Time: The new germ theory of disease*. New York: Anchor Books.

Eyler, John, 2010. 'The State of Science, Microbiology, and Vaccines Circa 1918', *Public Health Reports*, 125 Supp. 3: 27–36.

Faria, Nuno R., Andrew Rambaut, Marc A. Suchard, et al., 2014. 'HIV Epidemiology: The early spread and epidemic ignition of HIV-1 in human populations', *Science*, 346/6205: 56–61.

Farmer, Paul, 2003. *Pathologies of Power: Health, human*

rights, and the new war on the poor. Berkeley: University of California Press.

Farmer, Paul, 2014. 'Diary: Ebola', *London Review of Books*, 36.20, 23 October. https://www.lrb.co.uk/the-paper/v36/n20/paul-farmer/diary

FBI, 2010. 'Amerithrax or Anthrax Investigation', Washington, DC: FBI. https://www.fbi.gov/history/famous-cases/amerithrax-or-anthrax-investigation

Feachem, Richard, 1982. 'Environmental Aspects of Cholera Epidemiology. III. Transmission and control', *Tropical Diseases Bulletin*, 79: 1–47.

Ferguson, Neil, Daniel Laydon, Gemma Nadjati-Gilani, et al., 2020. 'Impact of Non-pharmaceutical Interventions (NPIs) to Reduce COVID-19 Mortality and Healthcare Demand', London: Imperial College COVID-19 Response Team, Report No. 9, 16 March.

Ferguson Niall, 1999. *The Pity of War: Explaining World War I*. London: Basic Books.

Ferguson, Niall, 2011. *Civilization: The West and the rest*. London: Allen Lane.

Fidler, David, 1999. *International Law and Infectious Diseases*. Oxford: Clarendon Press.

Fidler, David, 2003. 'SARS: Political Pathology of the First Post-Westphalian Pathogen', *The Journal of Law, Medicine and Ethics*, 31.4: 485–505.

Fidler, David, 2020. 'The World Health Organization and Pandemic Politics: The good, the bad, and an ugly future for global health', *Think Global Health*, 10 April. https://www.thinkglobalhealth.org/article/world-health-organization-and-pandemic-politics

Foss, Anna, Rachel von Simson, Cathy Zimmerman, et al., 2008. 'HIV/AIDS and Rape: Modelling predictions of the increase in individual risk of HIV infection from forced sex in conflict and post-conflict settings', New York: Social Science Research Council, HIV/AIDS, Security and Conflict Initiative Paper No. 24.

Fourie, Peter, and Martin Schönteich, 2001. 'Africa's New

Security Threat: HIV/AIDS and security in Southern Africa', *African Security Review*, 10.4: 29–44.

Frevert, Ute, 2009. 'German Conceptions of War, Masculinity and Femininity in the Long Nineteenth Century', in Sarah Colvin and Helen Watanabe-O'Kelly (eds), *Women and Death 2: Warlike women in the German literary and cultural imagination since 1500*. London: Camden House, pp. 169–85.

Fuks, Abraham, 2020. 'The Military Metaphors of Modern Medicine', in Zhenyi Li and Thomas Lawrence Long (eds), *The Meaning Management Challenge: Making sense of health, illness and disease*. Leiden: Brill, pp. 55–68.

Furmanski, Martin, 2014. 'Threatened Pandemics and Laboratory Escapes: Self-fulfilling prophecies', *Bulletin of the Atomic Scientists*, 31 March. https://thebulletin.org/2014/03/ threatened-pandemics-and-laboratory-escapes-self-fulfilling -prophecies/

Furmanski, Martin, 2015. 'The 1977 H1N1 Influenza Virus Reemergence Demonstrated Gain-of-Function Hazards', *mBio* 6.5: e01434-15. doi: 10.1128/mBio.01434-15

Garrett, Laurie, 1994. *The Coming Plague: Newly emerging diseases in a world out of balance*. New York: Farrar, Strauss & Giroux.

Garrett, Laurie, 2000. *Betrayal of Trust: The collapse of global public health*. New York: Hyperion Press.

Garrett, Laurie, 2005. 'We Are All Threatened by This Plague', International Herald Tribune, 29 July.

German Office of Sanitation, 2013, 'Influenza Mortality, German Armed Forces, 1917–1919', in Susan Kingsley Kent, *The Influenza Pandemic of 1918–1919: A brief history with documents*. Boston: Bedford/St Martin's, pp. 103–4.

Gibbon, Edward, 1782. *The History of the Decline and Fall of the Roman Empire*. London: Strahan.

Gisselquist, David, John Potterat, and Stuart Brody, 2003. 'Let It Be Sexual: How health care transmission of AIDS in Africa was ignored', *International Journal of STD and AIDS*, 14: 148–61.

Gomel, Elana, 2000. 'The Plague of Utopias: Pestilence and the apocalyptic body', *Twentieth-Century Literature*, 46.4: 405–33.

GPMB, 2019. 'A World at Risk: Annual report on global preparedness for health emergencies', Geneva: World Health Organization, Global Preparedness Monitoring Board, September.

GPMB, 2020. 'A World in Disorder: Annual report on global preparedness for health emergencies', Geneva: World Health Organization, Global Preparedness Monitoring Board, September.

Gradmann, Christoph, 2013. 'Exoticism, Bacteriology and the Staging of the Dangerous', in Thomas Rütter and Martina King (eds), *Contagionism and Contagious Diseases: Medicine and literature, 1880–1933*, Berlin: De Gruyter, pp. 65–82.

Grist, N.R., 1979. 'Pandemic Influenza 1918', *British Medical Journal*, 22 December: 1632–3.

Haacker, Marcus (ed.), 2004. *The Macroeconomics of HIV/AIDS.* Washington, DC: International Monetary Fund.

Hagemann, Karen, 1997. 'Of "Manly Valor" and "German Honor": Nation, war, and masculinity in the age of the Prussian uprising against Napoleon', *Central European History*, 30.2: 187–220.

Hamlin, Christopher, 2009. 'Commentary: Ackerknecht and "Anticontagionism": A tale of two dichotomies', *International Journal of Epidemiology*, 38: 22–7.

Hana, Emeline, Shu-Ti Chiou, Martin McKee, and Helena Legido-Quigley, 2020. 'The Resilience of Taiwan's Health System to Address the COVID-19 Pandemic', *Lancet*, 24/100437, June 26.

Hanna, Bridget, and Arthur Kleinman, 2013, 'Unpacking Global Health: Theory and critique', in Paul Farmer, Jim Yong Kim, Arthur Kleinman, and Matthew Basilico (eds), *Reimagining Global Health: An introduction.* Berkeley: University of California Press, pp. 15–32.

Hardy, Anne, 1993. 'Cholera, Quarantine and the English Preventive System, 1850–1895', *Medical History*, 37: 250–69.

Hatchett, Richard, Carter Mecher, and Marc Lipsitch, 2007. 'Public Health Interventions and Epidemic Intensity during the 1918 Influenza Pandemic', *Proceedings of the National Academy of Sciences* 104.18: 7582–7.

Hayden, Erika Check, 2011. 'The Price of Protection', *Nature*, 477: 150–3.

Henig, Robin Marantz, 1994. *A Dancing Matrix: How science confronts emerging viruses.* New York: Vintage.

Henze, Charlotte, 2011. *Disease, Health Care and Government in Late Imperial Russia: Life and death on the Volga, 1823–1914*, London: Routledge.

Heywood, Mark, 2005. 'Shaping, Making and Breaking the Law in the Campaign for a National HIV/AIDS Treatment Plan', in Peris Jones and Kristian Stokke (eds), *Democratising Development: The politics of socio-economic rights in South Africa.* Leiden: Martinus Nijhoff Publishers, pp. 101–22.

Holohan, Dan, 2017. *The Lost Art of Steam Heating, Revisited.* Scotts Valley, CA: CreateSpace.

Hooper, Edward, 1999. *The River: A journey to the source of HIV and AIDS.* London: Penguin.

Hoover, Irwin Hood, 2013. 'The Truth about Wilson's Illness, 1934', in Susan Kingsley Kent, *The Influenza Pandemic of 1918–1919: A brief history with documents.* Boston: Bedford/St Martin's.

Huang, Yanzhong, 2004. 'The SARS Epidemic and Its Aftermath in China: A political perspective', in Stacey Knobler, Adel Mahmoud, Stanley Lemon, Alison Mack, Laura Sivitz, and Katherine Oberholtzer (eds), *Learning from SARS: Preparing for the next disease outbreak.* Washington, DC: Institute of Medicine, pp. 116–32.

Huizinga, Johan, 1924. *The Waning of the Middle Ages*, translated by Frederick Hopman. London: Edward Arnold.

Humphries, Mark, 2014. 'Paths of Infection: The First World War and the origins of the 1918 influenza pandemic', *War in History*, 21.1: 55–81.

Hutchinson, Janis, 2003. 'HIV and the Evolution of Infectious Diseases', in George Ellison, Melissa Parker, and Catherine

Campbell (eds), *Learning from HIV and AIDS*. Cambridge: Cambridge University Press, pp. 32–58.

Imai, Masaki, Toiko Watanabe, Masato Hatta, et al., 2012. 'Experimental Adaptation of an Influenza H5 HA Confers Respiratory Droplet Transmission to a Reassortant H5 HA/H1N1 Virus in Ferrets', *Nature*, 486: 420–8.

Inglesby, Thomas, Jennifer Nuzzo, Tara O'Toole, and D. A. Henderson, 2006. 'Disease Mitigation Measures in the Control of Pandemic Influenza', *Biosecurity and Bioterrorism: Biodefense Strategy, Practice, and Science*, 4.4: 366–75.

Isabirye, Joel, 2008. 'Philly Lutaaya: Popular music and the fight against HIV/AIDS in Uganda', *Journal of Postcolonial Writing*, 44.1: 29–35.

Isherwood, Christopher, 2008. *The Berlin Stories*. New York: New Directions Books (originally published 1934).

Johns Hopkins, 2001. 'Dark Winter: Bioterrorism Exercise Andrews Air Force Base June 22–23, 2001', Baltimore, MD, and Washington, DC: Johns Hopkins Center for Civilian Biodefense, Center for Strategic and International Studies, ANSER, and Memorial Institute for the Prevention of Terrorism. https://www.centerforhealthsecurity.org/our-work/events-archive/2001_dark-winter/Dark%20Winter%20Script.pdf

Johns Hopkins Center for Health Security, 2019. 'Preparedness for a High-impact Respiratory Pathogen Pandemic', Baltimore, MD: Johns Hopkins Bloomberg School of Public Health.

Johnson, Steven, 2006. *The Ghost Map: The story of London's most terrifying epidemic – and how it changed sciences, cities, and the modern world*. New York: Riverhead.

Joint Learning Initiative on Children and HIV/AIDS, 2009. *Home Truths: Facing the facts on children, AIDS, and poverty*, Cambridge, MA: Harvard University, Global Equity Initiative.

Jordan, Douglas, with Terrence Tumpey and Barbara Jester, 2019. 'The Deadliest Flu: The complete story of the discovery and reconstruction of the 1918 pandemic virus',

Atlanta, GA: Centers for Disease Control and Prevention, https://www.cdc.gov/flu/pandemic-resources/reconstruction-1918-virus.html

Joyner, James, 2018. 'Bolton Dismantles White House Global Security Health Team', *Outside the Beltway*, 11 May. https://www.outsidethebeltway.com/bolton-dismantles-white-house-global-health-security-team/

Kaldor, Mary, 2012. *New and Old Wars: Organized violence in a global era*, Third edition. Cambridge: Polity.

Kamradt-Scott, Adam, 2015. *Managing Global Health Security: The World Health Organization and disease outbreak control.* London: Palgrave.

Kaplan, Robert, 1994. 'The Coming Anarchy: How crime, overpopulation, tribalism, and disease are rapidly destroying the social fabric of our planet', *Atlantic Monthly*, February.

Kaufman, Joan, 2005. 'SARS and China's Health-care Response: Better to be both red and expert!' in Arthur Kleinman and James Watson (eds), *SARS in China: Prelude to pandemic?* Stanford: Stanford University Press, pp. 53–70.

Kay, John, and Mervyn King, 2020. *Radical Uncertainty: Decision-making beyond the numbers.* New York: Norton.

Keller, Richard, 2006. 'Geographies of Power, Legacies of Mistrust: Colonial medicine and the global present', *Historical Geography*, 34: 26–48.

Kelly, Heath, 2011. 'The Classical Definition of a Pandemic Is Not Elusive', *Bulletin of the World Health Organization*, 89: 540–1.

Kent, Susan Kingsley, 2013, *The Influenza Pandemic of 1918–1919: A brief history with documents.* Boston: Bedford/St Martin's.

Kenyon, Chris, and Jozefien Buyze, 2015. 'No Association between Gender Inequality and Peak HIV Prevalence in Developing Countries: An ecological study', *AIDS Care*, 27:2: 150–9.

Killingray, David, 2003. 'A New "Imperial Disease": The influenza pandemic of 1918–19 and its impact on the British Empire', *Caribbean Quarterly*, 49.4: 30–49.

Kirchhoff, Christopher, 2016. 'NSC Lessons Learned Study on Ebola', Memorandum for Ambassador Susan E. Rice, 11 July. https://www.hsdl.org/?abstract&did=835350

Kleinman, Arthur, and James Watson, 2005. 'Introduction: SARS in social and historical context', in Arthur Kleinman and James Watson (eds), *SARS in China: Prelude to pandemic?* Stanford: Stanford University Press, pp. 1–16.

Klotz, Lynn, 2019. 'Human Error in High-biocontainment Labs: A likely pandemic threat', *Bulletin of the Atomic Scientists*, 25 February. https://thebulletin.org/2019/02/human-error-in-high-biocontainment-labs-a-likely-pandemic-threat/

Koblenz, Gregory, 2009. 'The Threat of Pandemic Influenza: Why today is not 1918', *World Medical and Health Policy*, 1.1: 71–84.

Kolko, Gabriel, 1994. *Century of War: Politics, conflicts, and society since 1914*. New York: The New Press.

Kraikovski, Alexei, 2013. 'The St Petersburg Cholera Riot of 1831: Water pollution and social tension'. Rachel Carson Center for Environment and Society Environment and Society Portal, *Arcadia* 9.

Krieger, Nancy, 2011. *Epidemiology and the People's Health: Theory and context*. New York: Oxford University Press.

Kuo, Steve, 2016. 'Taiwan's Role in War on Disease', *Taipei Times*, 1 June.

Kupferschmidt, Kai, 2015. 'Discovered a Disease? WHO has new rules for avoiding offensive names', *Science*, 11 May. https://www.sciencemag.org/news/2015/05/discovered-disease-who-has-new-rules-avoiding-offensive-names

Lakoff, Andrew, 2017. *Unprepared: Global health in a time of emergency*. Berkeley: University of California Press.

Larson, Heidi, 2020. *Stuck: How vaccine rumors start – and why they don't go away*. New York: Oxford University Press.

Latour, Bruno, 2017. *Facing Gaia: Eight lectures on the new climatic regime*, translated by Catherine Porter. Cambridge: Polity.

Lederberg, Joshua, Robert Shope, and Stanley Oaks (eds),

1992. *Emerging Infections: Microbial threats to health in the United States*. Washington, DC: Institute of Health.

Lee, Jong-Wha, and Warwick J. McKibbin, 2004. 'Estimating the Global Economic Costs of SARS', in Stacey Knobler, Adel Mahmoud, Stanley Lemon, Alison Mack, Laura Sivitz, and Katherine Oberholtzer (eds), *Learning from SARS: Preparing for the next disease outbreak*, Washington, DC: Institute of Medicine, pp. 91–109.

Lippi, D., and E. Gutozzo, 2014. 'The Greatest Steps towards the Discovery of *Vibrio cholerae*', *Clinical Microbiology and Infection*, 20.3: 191–5.

Lipton, Eric, and Jennifer Steinhauer, 2020. 'The Untold Story of the Birth of Social Distancing', *New York Times*, 22 April. https://www.nytimes.com/2020/04/22/us/politics/social-distancing-coronavirus.html

Lucas, Sebastian, 2000. 'The River: A journey back to the source of HIV and AIDS', *British Medical Journal*, 320/7247: 1481A.

Lynteris, Christos, 2016. 'Untimely Ends and the Pandemic Imaginary', *Somatosphere*, 8 July. http://somatosphere.net/2016/untimely-ends-and-the-pandemic-imaginary.html/

Machel, Samora, 1975. *Mozambique: Sowing the seeds of revolution*. London: Committee for Freedom in Mozambique, Angola, and Guinea.

MacMillan, Margaret, 2003. *Paris 1919: Six months that changed the world*. New York: Random House.

Maglen, Krista, 2002. '"The First Line of Defence": British quarantine and the port sanitary authorities in the nineteenth century', *Social History of Medicine*, 15.3: 413–28.

Mann, Jonathan, Lawrence Gostin, Sofia Gruskin, et al. 1994. 'Health and Human Rights', *Health and Human Rights*, 1.1: 6–23.

Markel, Howard, 1995. 'Knocking out the Cholera: Cholera, class, and quarantines in New York City, 1892', *Bulletin of the History of Medicine*, 69.3: 420–57.

Markel, Howard, Alexandra Stern, Alexander Navarro, et al.,

2006. 'Nonpharmaceutical Influenza Mitigation Strategies, US Communities, 1918–1920 Pandemic', *Emerging Infectious Diseases*, 12.12: 1961–5.

Markel, Howard, Harvey Lipman, Alexander Navarro, et al., 2007. 'Nonpharmaceutical Interventions Implemented by US Cities During the 1918-1919 Influenza Pandemic', *Journal of the American Medical Association*, 298.6: 644–55.

Martin, Andrew, and Clifford Krauss, 2009. 'Pork Industry Fights Concerns over Swine Flu', *New York Times*, 28 April. https://www.nytimes.com/2009/04/29/business/economy/29trade.html

Mayhew, Robert, 2014. *Malthus*. Cambridge, MA: Harvard University Press.

Mbali, Mandisa, 2005. 'The Treatment Action Campaign and the History of Rights-based, Patient-driven HIV/AIDS Activism in South Africa', in Peris Jones and Kristian Stokke (eds), *Democratising Development: The politics of socio-economic rights in South Africa*. Leiden: Martinus Nijhoff Publishers, pp. 213–44.

McClenna, Ely, 1885. 'Cholera Hygiene as Applied to Military Life', in Edmund Charles Wendt (ed.), *A Treatise on Asiatic Cholera*. New York: William Wood, pp. 71–118.

McDonald, J.C., 1951. 'The History of Quarantine in Britain during the 19th Century', *Bulletin of the History of Medicine*, 25.1: 22–44.

McGrew, R.E., 1960. 'The First Cholera Epidemic and Social History', *Bulletin of the History of Medicine*, 34.1: 61–73.

McNeill, William H., 1977. *Plagues and Peoples*. New York: Anchor Books.

McPherson, Malcolm, Deborah Hoover, and Donald Snodgrass, 2000. 'The Impact on Economic Growth in Africa of Rising Costs and Labor Productivity Losses Associated with HIV/AIDS', Cambridge, MA: JFK School of Government, Harvard, August.

Mehra, Akhil, 2009. 'Politics of Participation: Walter Reed's yellow-fever experiments', *American Medical Association Journal of Ethics*, 11.4: 326–30.

Meltzer, M.I., C.Y. Atkins, S. Santibanez, et al. 2014. 'Estimating the Future Number of Cases in the Ebola Epidemic – Liberia and Sierra Leone, 2014–2015', *MMWR Suppl.* 63.3: 1-14.

Meltzer M.I., S. Santibanez, L.S. Fischer, et al. 2016. 'Modeling in Real Time during the Ebola Response', *MMWR Suppl* 65 Supplement 3: 85–9.

Moon S., D. Sridhar, M.A. Pate, et al. 2015. 'Will Ebola Change the Game? Ten essential reforms before the next pandemic. The report of the Harvard–LSHTM Independent Panel on the Global Response to Ebola', *Lancet*, 386: 2204–21.

Morabia, Alfredo, 2007. 'Epidemiologic Interactions, Complexity, and the Lonesome Death of Max von Pettenkofer', *American Journal of Epidemiology*, 166.11: 1233–8.

Morens, David, and Anthony Fauci, 2020. 'Emerging Pandemic Diseases: How we got to COVID-19', *Cell*, 182: 1077–92.

Morens, David, and Jeffery K. Taubenberger, 2010. 'Historical Thoughts on Influenza Viral Ecosystems, or Behold a Pale Horse, Dead Dogs, Failing Fowl, and Sick Swine', *Influenza and Other Respiratory Viruses*, 4: 327–37.

Morens, David, and Jeffery Taubenberger, 2011. 'Pandemic Influenza: Certain uncertainties', *Reviews in Medical Virology*, 21: 262–84.

Morens, David, Jeffery Taubenberger, and Anthony Fauci, 2009. 'The Persistent Legacy of the 1918 Influenza Virus', *New England Journal of Medicine*, 361.3: 225–9.

Morner, Andrew, and Michel Garenne, 2000. 'The 1918 Influenza Epidemic's Effects on Sex Differentials in Mortality in the United States', *Population and Development Review*, 26.3: 565–81.

Morris, Martina, and Mirjam Kretzschmar, 1997. 'Concurrent Partnerships and the Spread of HIV', *AIDS*, 11.5: 641–8.

Mullet, Mary B., 1918. 'The Chances of Getting Killed or Hurt in This War: An important message to *American*

Magazine readers from Surgeon General Gorgas', *American Magazine*, 85, March: 41–3.

Murray, Christopher, 2020. 'Coronavirus Crisis Update: Dr Christopher Murray on the "Chris Murray Model"', Center for Strategic and International Studies podcast, *Take as Directed*, 15 April. https://www.csis.org/podcasts/take-directed-coronavirus-crisis-update

Musk, Matthew, 2020. 'George W. Bush in 2005: "If we wait for a pandemic to appear, it will be too late to prepare"', ABC News, 5 April. https://abcnews.go.com/Politics/george-bush-2005-wait-pandemic-late-prepare/story?id=69979013

Nagel, Thomas, 1974. 'What Is It Like to Be a Bat?' *Philosophical Review*, 83.4: 435–50.

National Hog Farmer, 2009. 'Swine Flu Officially Changed to "2009 H1N1 Flu"', *National Hog Farmer*, 30 April.

National Intelligence Council, 2000. 'The Global Infectious Disease Threat and Its Implications for the United States'. Washington, DC: NIC, NIE 99-17D, January.

National Intelligence Council, 2002. 'The Next Wave of HIV/AIDS: Nigeria, Ethiopia, Russia, India, and China', Washington, DC: NIC, ICA 2002-04 D, September.

National Intelligence Council, 2008. 'Strategic implications of Global Health'. Washington, DC: NIC, ICA 2008-10D, December.

Neilson, Trevor, 2005. 'AIDS, Economics and Terrorism in Africa', London: Global Business Coalition on AIDS, January.

Nie, Jing-Bao, 1996. 'The Physician as General', *Journal of the American Medical Association*. 279.13: 1099. doi: 10.1001/jama.276.13.1099. PMID: 8847777.

Nie, Jing-Bao, Adam Lloyd Gilbertson, Malcolm de Roubaix, et al., 2016. 'Healing without Waging War: Beyond military metaphors in medicine and HIV cure research', *American Journal of BioEthics*, 16.10, 3–11.

Normile, Dennis, 2005. 'Pandemic Skeptics Warn against Crying Wolf', *Science* 310/5751: 1112–13.

North, Douglass, 1991. 'Institutions', *Journal of Economic Perspectives*, 5.1: 97–112.

Obbo, Christine, 1993. 'HIV Transmission through Social and Geographical Networks in Uganda', *Social Science and Medicine*, 36: 949–55.

Ondoga ori Amaza, 1998. *Museveni's Long March from Guerrilla to Statesman*. Kampala: Fountain Press.

Onion, Rebecca, 2020. 'The 1918 Flu Pandemic Killed Millions. So why does its cultural memory feel so faint?' *Slate*, 3 May. https://slate.com/human-interest/2020/05/1918-pandemic-cultural-memory-literature-outka.html

Oppenheimer, Gerald M., and Ezra Susser, 2007. 'Invited Commentary: The context and challenge of von Pettenkofer's contributions to epidemiology', *American Journal of Epidemiology*, 166.11: 1239–41.

Osane, Olivia, 2018. 'Humans and Big Ag Livestock Now Account for 96 Percent of Mammal Biomass', *Ecowatch*, 23 May. https://www.ecowatch.com/biomass-humans-animals-2571413930.html

Osler, William, 1914. 'Bacilli and Bullets: An address to the officers and men in the camps at Churn', *British Medical Journal*, 3 October: 569–70.

Osterholm, Michael, 2005. 'Prepared Statement', Testimony before the House Committee on International Relations, 'Avian Flu: Addressing the global threat', Washington, DC, 7 December. https://www.govinfo.gov/content/pkg/CHRG-109hhrg24906/pdf/CHRG-109hhrg24906.pdf

Osterholm, Michael, 2020. 'A Tale of Two Countries', *The Osterholm Update: COVID-19*, Minneapolis: University of Minnesota, Center for Infectious Disease Research and Policy, 17 June. https://www.cidrap.umn.edu/covid-19/podcasts-webinars/episode-12

Osterholm, Michael, and Mark Olshaker, 2017. *Deadliest Enemy: Our war against killer germs*. New York: Little Brown Spark.

O'Toole, Tara, Mair Michael, and Thomas V. Inglesby,

2002. 'Shining Light on "Dark Winter"', *Clinical Infectious Diseases*, 34.7: 972–83.

Outka, Elizabeth, 2019. *Viral Modernism: The influenza pandemic and interwar literature.* New York: Columbia University Press.

Oxford, John S., 2001, 'The So-called Great Spanish Influenza Pandemic of 1918 May Have Originated in France in 1916', *Philosophical Transactions of the Royal Society of London B: Biological Science*, 356: 1857–9.

Oxford, John S., and Douglas Gill, 2019. 'A Possible European Origin of the Spanish Influenza and the First Attempts to Reduce Mortality to Combat Superinfecting Bacteria: An opinion from a virologist and a military historian', *Human Vaccines and Immunotherapeutics*, 15.9: 2009–12.

Parker, Melissa, Tommy Matthew Hanson, Ahmed Vandi, Lawrence Sao Babawo, and Tim Allen, 2019. 'Ebola and Public Authority: Saving loved ones in Sierra Leone', *Medical Anthropology*, 38.5: 440–54.

Paxton, Nathan, 2014. 'Plague, War, and Democracy: Political processes and the spread of HIV', *Social Science Research Network*, 16. http://dx.doi.org/10.2139/ssrn.2416896

Peckham, Robert, 2016. 'Where Has SARS Gone? The strange case of the disappearing coronavirus', *Somatosphere*, 8 June. http://somatosphere.net/2016/where-has-sars-gone -the-strange-case-of-the-disappearing-coronavirus.html/

Peikoff, Leonard, 1991. *Objectivism: The philosophy of Ayn Rand.* New York: Meridian.

Pepin, Jacques, 2011. *The Origins of AIDS.* Cambridge: Cambridge University Press.

Perrow, Charles, 1984. *Normal Accidents: Living with high-risk technologies*, New York: Basic Books.

Peters, F.E., 1994. *The Hajj: The Muslim pilgrimage to Mecca and the Holy Places.* Princeton: Princeton University Press.

Peters, John, 1885. 'General History of the Disease and the Principal Epidemics up to 1885', in Edmund Charles Wendt (ed.), *A Treatise on Asiatic Cholera.* New York: William Wood, pp. 3–70.

Petro, Anthony, 2015. *After the Wrath of God: AIDS, sexuality, and American religion.* Oxford: Oxford University Press.

Pharoah, Robyn (ed.), 2004. *A Generation at Risk? HIV/AIDS, Vulnerable children and security in southern Africa.* Pretoria: Institute for Security Studies.

Phillips, Howard, 1990. *'Black October': The impact of the Spanish influenza epidemic of 1918 on South Africa.* Archive Yearbook of South African History, 53, 1. Pretoria: The Government Printer.

Phillips, Howard, 2004. 'The Re-appearing Shadow of 1918: Trends in the historiography of the 1918–19 influenza pandemic', *Canadian Bulletin of Medical History*, 21.1: 121–34.

Pinkard, Terry, 2000. *Hegel: A biography.* Cambridge: Cambridge University Press.

Piot, Peter, 2012. *No Time to Lose: A life in pursuit of deadly viruses.* New York: Norton.

Piot, Peter, Francis Plummer, Marie-Anne Rey, et al., 1987. 'Retrospective Seroepidemiology of AIDS Virus Infection in Nairobi Populations', *Journal of Infectious Diseases*, 155: 1108–12.

Piper, Kelsey, 2020 'Why Some Labs Work on Making Viruses Deadlier – and why they should stop', *Vox*, 1 May. https://www.vox.com/2020/5/1/21243148/why-some-labs-work-on-making-viruses-deadlier-and-why-they-should-stop

Pisani, Elizabeth, 2008. *The Wisdom of Whores: Bureaucrats, brothels and the business of AIDS.* New York: W.W. Norton.

Plowright, Raina, Patrick Foley, Hume Field, et al., 2011. 'Urban Habituation, Ecological Connectivity and Epidemic Dampening: The emergence of Hendra Virus in flying foxes (*Pteropus spp.*)', *Proceedings of the Royal Society B*, 278: 3703–12.

Pomfret, John, 2003. 'Outbreak Gave China's Hu an Opening', *Washington Post*, 13 May.

President of the United States, 2010. *National Security Strategy*, Washington, DC: The White House, May.

Preston, Richard, 1994. *The Hot Zone: The terrifying true story of the origins of the Ebola virus.* New York: Anchor Books.

Pullan, Brian, 1992. 'Plague and Perceptions of the Poor in Early Modern Italy', in Terence Ranger and Paul Slack (eds), *Epidemics and Ideas: Essays on the historical perception of pestilence*. Cambridge: Cambridge University Press, pp. 101–24.

Quammen, David, 2012. *Spillover: Animal infections and the next human pandemic*. New York: Norton.

Racaniello, Vincent, 2016. 'Dugas was Not Patient Zero', Virology Blog, 16 November. https://www.virology.ws/2016/11/16/dugas-was-not-aids-patient-zero/

Racaniello, Vincent, 2020. 'The SARS-CoV-2 Pandemic Could Have Been Prevented', Virology Blog, 30 April. https://www.virology.ws/2020/04/30/the-sars-cov-2-pandemic-could-have-been-prevented/

Raguin, G., A. Lepretre, I. Ba, I. Ndoye, A. Toufik, G. Brucker, and P.-M. Girard, 2011. 'Drug Use and HIV in West Africa: A neglected epidemic', *Tropical Medicine & International Health*, 16: 1131–3.

Rand, Ayn, 1999. *The Return of the Primitive: The anti-industrial revolution*, edited with an introduction and additional essays by Peter Schwartz. Harmondsworth: Penguin.

Ranger, Terence, 1992. 'Plagues of Beasts and Men: Prophetic responses to epidemic in eastern and southern Africa', in Terence Ranger and Paul Slack (eds), *Epidemics and Ideas: Essays on the historical perception of pestilence*. Cambridge: Cambridge University Press, pp. 241–68.

Reid, Ann H., Thomas G. Fanning, Johan V. Hultin, and Jeffery K. Taubenberger, 1999. 'Origin and Evolution of the 1918 "Spanish" Influenza Virus Hemagglutinin Gene', *Proceedings of the National Academy of Sciences*, 96.4: 1651–6.

Reid, Anne H., Thomas G. Fanning, Thomas A. Janczewski, and Jeffery K. Taubenberger, 2000. 'Characterization of the 1918 "Spanish Influenza" Virus Neuraminidase Gene', *Proceedings of the National Academy of Sciences*, 97.12: 6785–90.

Rhodes, Richard, 1986. *The Making of the Atomic Bomb*. New York: Simon & Schuster.

Ribacke, Kim Brolin, Dell Saulnier, Anneli Eriksson, and Johan von Schreeb, 2016. 'Effects of the West Africa Ebola Virus Disease on Health-Care Utilization: A systematic review', *Frontiers in Public Health*, 10 October. doi: 10.3389/fpubh.2016.00222

Richards, Paul, 2016. *Ebola: How a people's science helped end an epidemic*. London, Zed Books.

Rosner, David, 2010. '"Spanish Flu, or Whatever It Is. . . .": The paradox of public health in a time of crisis', *Public Health Reports*, 125 Supplement 3: 38–48.

Ross, Richard, 2015. *Contagion in Prussia, 1831: The cholera epidemic and the threat of the Polish uprising.* Jefferson, NC: MacFarland.

Rothfels, Hans, 1943. 'Clausewitz', in Edwin Meade Earle (ed.), *Makers of Modern Strategy: Military Thought from Machiavelli to Hitler.* Princeton: Princeton University Press.

Rozo, Michele, and Gigi Kwik Gronvall, 2015. 'The Reemergent 1977 H1N1 Strain and the Gain-of-Function Debate', *mBio* 6:e01013-15. doi: 10.1128/mBio.01013-15

Rumsfeld, Donald, 2002. 'Department of Defense Briefing', 12 February. https://www.nato.int/docu/speech/2002/s020606g.htm

Saich, Tony, 2005. 'China's Chernobyl or Much Ado about Nothing?', in Arthur Kleinman and James Watson (eds), *SARS in China: Prelude to pandemic?* Stanford: Stanford University Press, pp. 71–104.

Saich, Tony, 2020. 'Tony Saich on China's Leadership during the COVID-19 Outbreak', Harvard Kennedy School, Ash Center. https://ash.harvard.edu/tony-saich-china%E2%80%99s-leadership-during-covid-19-outbreak?admin_panel=1

Sands, Peter, Anas El Turabi, Philip Saynisch, and Victor Dzau, 2016. 'Assessment of Economic Vulnerability to Infectious Disease Crises', *Lancet* 388: 2443–8.

Sartin, Jeffrey, 1993. 'Infectious Diseases during the Civil War: The triumph of the "Third Army"', *Clinical Infectious Diseases*, 16.4: 580–4.

Sauter, Daniel, and Frank Kirchhoff, 2019. 'Key Viral Adaptations Preceding the AIDS Pandemic', *Cell Host and Microbe*, 25.1: 27–38.

Schlosser, Eric, 2013. *Command and Control: Nuclear weapons, the Damascus incident, and the illusion of safety*. New York: Penguin.

Schnirring, Lisa, 2017. 'Feds Lift Gain-of-Function Research Pause, Offer Guidance', CIDRAP News, 19 December. https://www.cidrap.umn.edu/news-perspective/2017/12/feds -lift-gain-function-research-pause-offer-guidance

Schönteich, Martin, 2000. 'Age and AIDS: South Africa's crime time bomb', Pretoria: Institute for Security Studies.

Scoones, Ian, 2020, 'Science, Uncertainty and the COVID-19 Response', STEPS Centre, 16 March. https://steps-centre. org/blog/science-uncertainty-and-the-covid-19-response

Scoones, Ian, K. Jones, G. Lo Iacono, et al., 2017. 'Integrative Modelling for One Health: Pattern, process and participation', *Philosophical Transactions of the Royal Society B*: 372: 20160164. doi: 10.1098/rstb.2016.0164

Seaman, Rebecca, 2018. 'Cholera: Dread disease of the Crimean War, 1954–1855', in Rebecca Seaman (ed.), *Epidemics and War: The impact of disease on major conflicts in history*. Santa Barbara, CA: ABC-CLIO, pp. 83–96.

Segal, David, 2020. 'Why Are There Almost No Memorials to the Flu of 1918?', *New York Times*, 14 May. https:// www.nytimes.com/2020/05/14/business/1918-flu-memorial s.html?

Semino, Elena, Zsófia Demjén, Andrew Hardie, Sheila Payne, and Paul Rayson, 2018. *Metaphor, Cancer and the End of Life: A corpus-based study*. New York: Routledge.

Senior Curate of St Luke's [Henry Whitehead], 1854. *The Cholera in Berwick Street*. London: Hope & Co. http://kora. matrix.msu.edu/files/21/120/15-78-7C-22-1854-10-White head.PDF

Shell, Robert, 1999. 'The Silent Revolution: The AIDS pandemic and the military in South Africa', in Konrad Adenauer

Foundation, *Consolidating Democracy in South Africa*. East London: Konrad Adenauer Foundation, pp. 29–41.

Shilts, Randy, 1987. *And the Band Played On: Politics, people and the AIDS epidemic*. New York: St Martin's Press.

Shoumatoff, Alex, 1988. 'In Search of the Source of AIDS', *Vanity Fair*, July.

Skulls in the Stars, 2014. 'The Great Sausage Duel of 1865', *Skulls in the Stars*, 1 November. https://skullsinthestars.com/2014/11/01/the-great-sausage-duel-of-1865/

Slack, Paul, 1992. 'Introduction', in Terence Ranger and Paul Slack (eds), *Epidemics and Ideas: Essays on the historical perception of pestilence*. Cambridge: Cambridge University Press, pp. 1–20.

Smallman-Raynor, M.R., and A.D. Cliff, 2004. *War Epidemics: An historical geography of infectious diseases in military conflict and civil strife, 1850–2000*. Oxford: Oxford University Press.

Smith, Adrian, Placide Tapsoba, Norbert Peshu, Eduard Sanders, and Harold Jaffe, 2009. 'Men Who Have Sex with Men and HIV/AIDS in Sub-Saharan Africa', *The Lancet*, 374/9687: 416–22.

Smith, Geddes, 1943. *Plague on Us*. New York: The Commonwealth Fund.

Snacken, René, Alan P. Kendal, Lars R. Haaheim, and John M. Wood, 1999. 'The Next Influenza Pandemic: Lessons from Hong Kong, 1997', *Emerging Infectious Diseases*, 5.2: 195–203.

Sontag, Susan, 1988. *Illness as Metaphor and AIDS and Its Metaphors*. New York: Picador.

Spellberg, Brad, and Bonnie Taylor-Blake, 2013. 'On the Exoneration of Dr William H. Stewart: Debunking an urban legend', *Infectious Diseases of Poverty*, 2.3. doi: 10.1186/2049-9957-2-3

Spiegel, Paul, 2004. 'HIV/AIDS among Conflict-affected and Displaced Populations', *Disasters*, 28: 322–39.

Spinney, Laura, 2017. *Pale Rider: The Spanish Flu of 1918 and how it changed the world*. New York: Public Affairs.

Stach, Reiner, 2013. *Kafka: The years of insight*, translated by Shelley Frisch. Princeton: Princeton University Press.

Stefanou-Konidaris, Natasha, 2020. 'Letter: Virus offers opportunity to fix linguistic anomaly', *Financial Times*, 3 May.

Stern, Alexandra Minna, 2006. 'Yellow Fever Crusade: US colonialism, tropical medicine, and the international politics of mosquito control, 1900–1920', in Alison Bashford (ed.), *Medicine at the Border: Disease, globalization and security, 1850 to the present*. London: Palgrave, pp. 41–59.

Strathdee, Steffanie, and Jamila Stockman, 2010. 'Epidemiology of HIV among Injecting and Non-injecting Drug Users: Current trends and implications for intervention', *Current HIV/AIDS Reports*, 7: 99–106.

Supervie, Virginie, Yasmin Halima, and Sally Blower, 2010. 'Assessing the Impact of Mass Rape on the Incidence of HIV in Conflict-affected Countries', *AIDS*, 24.18: 2841–7.

Tamale, Sylvia (ed.), 2011. *African Sexualities: A reader*. London: Pambazuka Press.

Taubenberger, Jeffery, Ann Reid, Amy Krafft, Karen Bijwaard, and Thomas Fanning, 1997. 'Initial Genetic Characterization of the 1918 "Spanish" Influenza Virus', *Science* 21: 1793–6.

Thompson, James, 1921. 'The Aftermath of the Black Death and the Aftermath of the Great War', *American Journal of Sociology*, 26.5: 565–72.

Tilly, Charles, 1990. *Coercion, Capital and European States, AD 990–1992*. Oxford: Blackwell.

Tomes, Nancy, 2010. '"Destroyer and Teacher": Managing the masses during the 1918–1919 influenza pandemic', *Public Health Reports*, 125 Supplement 3: 48–62.

Tompa, Rachel, 2017. 'Understanding HIV's Evolutionary Past – and Future', Fred Hutch News Service, 20 November. https://www.fredhutch.org/en/news/center-news/2017/11/hiv-evolutionary-past-and-future.html

Tuchman, Barbara, 1979. *A Distant Mirror: The calamitous 14th century*. Harmondsworth: Penguin.

Tumpey, Terrence M., Christopher F. Baster, Patricia V. Aguilar, et al. 2005. 'Characterization of the Reconstructed 1918 Spanish Influenza Pandemic Virus', *Science*. 310/5745: 77–80.

Tumushabe, Joseph, 2005. 'The Politics of HIV/AIDS in Uganda', Geneva: UN Research Institute for Social Development, July.

Twain, Mark, 1923. 'The Cholera Epidemic in Hamburg', in *The Writings of Mark Twain, Volume XXIX: Europe and Elsewhere*. New York: Gabriel Wells, pp. 186–92.

UN Theme Group on HIV/AIDS and China, 2002. *HIV/AIDS: China's Titanic Peril, 2001 Update of the AIDS Situation and Needs Assessment Report*. Geneva: UNAIDS.

UNAIDS, 1998. 'AIDS and the Military: UNAIDS point of view', Geneva: UNAIDS Best Practice Collection, May.

UNECA, 2001. 'Popular Report: African Development Forum 2000: Leadership at all levels to overcome HIV/AIDS'. Addis Ababa: UN Economic Commission for Africa.

University of Wisconsin-Madison, 2012. 'After Epic Debate, Avian Flu Research Sees Light of Day', *ScienceDaily*, 2 May. http://www.sciencedaily.com/releases/2012/05/120502143852.htm

Van Griensven, Fritz, 2007. 'Men Who have Sex with Men and Their HIV Epidemics in Africa', *AIDS*, 21: 1361–2.

Vandegrift, Kurt, Susanne Sokolow, Peter Daszak, and Marm Kilpatrick, 2010. 'Ecology of Avian Influenza Viruses in a Changing World', *Annals of the New York Academy of Sciences*, 1195: 113–28.

Vaughan, Megan, 1991. *Curing Their Ills: Colonial power and African illness*. Stanford: Stanford University Press.

Velmet, Aro, 2020. *Pasteur's Empire: Bacteriology and politics in France, its colonies, and the world*. Oxford: Oxford University Press.

Virchow, Rudolph, 1985. 'Report on the Typhus Epidemic in Upper Silesia', in *Collected Essays on Public Health and Epidemiology*, Vol. 1, edited by L.J. Rather. Boston: Science History Publications, pp. 204–319.

Wald, Priscilla, 2008. *Contagious: Cultures, carriers and the outbreak narrative*. Durham, NC: Duke University Press.

Walsh, Sinead, and Oliver Johnson, 2018. *Getting to Zero: A doctor and a diplomat on the Ebola frontline*. London: Zed Books.

Walter, Edward, and Mike Scott, 2017. 'The Life and Work of Rudolf Virchow 1821–1902: "Cell theory, thrombosis and the sausage duel"', *Journal of the Intensive Care Society*, 18.3: 234–5.

Watterson, Christopher, and Adam Kamradt-Scott, 2016. 'Fighting Flu: Securitization and the military role in combating influenza', *Armed Forces and Society*, 42.1: 145–68.

Watts, Charlotte, Cathy Zimmerman, Anna M. Foss, Mazeda Hossain, Andrew Cox, and Peter Vickerman, 2010. 'Remodelling Core Group Theory: The role of sustaining populations in HIV transmission', *Sexually Transmitted Infections*, 86 Supp.: iii85–92.

Watts, Sheldon, 1997. *Epidemics and History: Disease, power and imperialism*. New Haven: Yale University Press.

Watts, Sheldon, 2001. 'From Rapid Change to Stasis: Official responses to cholera in British-ruled India and Egypt: 1860 to c. 1921', *Journal of World History*, 12.2: 321–74.

Wertheim, Joel, 2010. 'The Re-emergence of H1N1 Influenza Virus in 1977: A cautionary tale for estimating divergence times using biologically unrealistic sampling dates', *PLoS ONE*, 5.6: e11184.

Wever, Peter C., and Leo van Bergen, 2014. 'Death from 1918 Pandemic Influenza during the First World War: A perspective from personal and anecdotal evidence', *Influenza and Other Respiratory Viruses*, 8.5: 538–46.

White, Luise, 1990. *The Comforts of Home: Prostitution in colonial Nairobi*. Chicago: University of Chicago Press.

Whiteside, Alan, 2008. *HIV & AIDS: A very short introduction*. Oxford: Oxford University Press.

Whiteside, Alan and Alex de Waal, 2003. 'New Variant Famine: AIDS and food crisis in southern Africa', *The Lancet*, 362/9391: 1234–7.

Whiteside, Alan, Robert Mattes, Samantha Willan, and Ryann Manning, 2003. 'Examining HIV/AIDS in Southern Africa through the Eyes of Ordinary Southern Africans', Cape Town: Afrobarometer Working Paper, No. 21.

Whiteside, Alan, Alex de Waal, and Tsadkan Gebre Tensae, 2006. 'AIDS, the Military and Security in Africa: A sober appraisal', *African Affairs*, 105/419: 201–8.

WHO, 1997. *EMC Annual Report 1997*. Geneva: WHO, Division of Emerging and Other Communicable Diseases Surveillance and Control.

WHO, 1998. 'Emerging Infectious Diseases: Memorandum from a WHO meeting', *Bulletin of the World Health Organization*, 76: 539–44.

WHO, 2015. 'WHO Issues Best Practices for Naming New Human Infectious Diseases', 8 May. https://www.who.int/mediacentre/news/notes/2015/naming-new-diseases/en/

WHO, 2018. 'Annual Review of Diseases Prioritized under the Research and Development Blueprint', Informal consultation, 6–7 February. https://www.who.int/docs/default-source/blue-print/2018-annual-review-of-diseases-prioritiz ed-under-the-research-and-development-blueprint.pdf?sfvr sn=4c22e36_2

Wilkinson, Eduan, Susan Engelbrecht, and Tulio de Oliveira, 2015. 'History and Origin of the HIV-1 Subtype C Epidemic in South Africa and the Greater Southern African Region', *Science Reports*, 5: 16897.

Wills, Christopher, 1996. *Yellow Fever, Black Goddess: The coevolution of people and plagues*. Reading MA: Helix Books.

Wootton, David, 2006. *Bad Medicine: Doctors doing harm since Hippocrates*. Oxford: Oxford University Press.

World Bank, 1999. *Confronting AIDS: Public priorities in a global epidemic*. Washington, DC: World Bank.

Worobey, Michael, Thomas Watts, Richard McKay, et al. 2016. '1970s and "Patient 0" HIV-1 Genomes Illuminate Early HIV/AIDS History in North America', *Nature* 539: 98–101.

Xiang, Biao, 2020. 'From Chain Reaction to Grid Reaction:

Mobilities and restrictions during the epidemics of SARS and COVID-19', *Somatosphere*, 6 March. http://somato sphere.net/forumpost/from-chain-to-grid-reaction/

XinuaNet, 2020. 'Xi Focus: Chronicle of Xi's leadership in China's war against coronavirus'. http://www.xinhuanet. com/english/2020-09/07/c_139349538.htm

Yang, Zheng, 2020. 'Military Metaphors in Contemporary Chinese Disease Coverage: A case study of the *People's Daily*, 1946–2019', *Chinese Journal of Communication*. doi: 10.1080/17544750.2020.1818593

Yeager, Roger, Craig Hendrix, and Stuart Kingma, 2000. 'International Military Human Immunodeficiency Virus/ Acquired Immunodeficiency Syndrome Policies and Programs: Strengths and limitations in current practice', *Military Medicine*, 165: 87–92.

Yebra, Gonzalo, Manon Ragonnet-Cronin, Deogratius Seemwanga, et al., 2015. 'Analysis of the History and Spread of HIV-1 in Uganda Using Phylodynamics', *The Journal of General Virology*, 96.7: 1890–8.

Zhang, Hong, 2005. 'Making Light of the Dark Side: SARS jokes and humor in China', in Arthur Kleinman and James Watson (eds), *SARS in China: Prelude to Pandemic?* Stanford: Stanford University Press, pp. 148–72.

Ziegler, Philip, 1969. *The Black Death*. London: Collins.

Zinsser, Hans, 1935. *Rats, Lice and History*. London: Routledge.

Zylberman, Patrick, 2007. 'Civilizing the State: Borders, weak states and international health in modern Europe', in Alison Bashford (ed.), *Medicine at the Border: Disease, globalization and security, 1850 to the present*. London: Palgrave, pp. 21–40.

Index